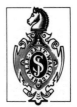

M. Castegnaro E. B. Sansone

Chemical Carcinogens

Some Guidelines for Handling and
Disposal in the Laboratory

Springer-Verlag Berlin Heidelberg New York
London Paris Tokyo

Dr. Marcel Castegnaro

International Agency for Research on Cancer
Unit of Environmental Carcinogens and Host Factors
150 Cours Albert-Thomas
F-69372 Lyon Cedex 08

Dr. Eric B. Sansone

Environmental Control & Research Program
NCI-Frederick Cancer Research Facility
Program Resources Inc.
P.O. Box B
Frederick, MD 21701/USA

ISBN 3-540-16719-6 Springer-Verlag Berlin Heidelberg New York
ISBN 0-387-16719-6 Springer-Verlag New York Heidelberg Berlin

Library of Congress Cataloging in Publication Data.
Castegnaro, M. (Marcel), 1944– Chemical carcinogens.
Bibliography: p.
1. Carcinogens – Safety measures. I. Sansone, E. B. (Eric Brandfon), 1939–. II. Title.
RC 268.6.C 38 1986 604.7 86-13921
ISBN 0-387-16719-6 (U.S.)

Typesetting: Hagedorn, Berlin; Offsetprinting: Heenemann, Berlin;
Bookbinding: Lüderitz & Bauer, Berlin
2152/3020–543210

After review of the various safety aspects related to the handling, storage, transportation of chemical carcinogens, the minimum requirements for installing a room where these substances can be stored and handled in bulk quantities are presented.

The various techniques of dispoal of wastes contaminated with chemical carcinogens are then discussed and some validated chemical degradation methods presented for the treatment of wastes and spillage containing aflatoxins, N-nitrosamines, N-nitrosamides, polycyclic aromatic hydrocarbons, hydrazines, aromatic amines, haloethers and some antineoplastic agents.

This research has been sponsored in part by the National Cancer Institute under Contract No. N01-CO-23910 with Program Resources Inc. and Contract No. 1-DS-2-2130 with the International Agency for Research on Cancer. The contents of this publication do not necessarily reflect the views or policies of the DHHS, nor does mention of trade names, commercial products, or organizations imply endorsement by the US Government.

Contents

List of Symbols and Abbreviations

IARC,   International Agency for Research for Cancer

NIH,   National Institute of Health (USA)

OSHA,   Occupational Safety and Health Administration (USA)

PAH,   polycyclic aromatic hydrocarbons

MOCA,   4,4'-methylene bis(2-chloroaniline)

1 Introduction

"The chemical laboratory is actually not a dangerous place to work in, but it demands a reasonable prudence on the part of the experimenters and instructers, to keep it a safe place. Emphasis must be positive, indicating the proper, correct and safe procedure to be followed in all laboratory operations or when confronted with an emergency situation. Too heavy stress upon the horrors associated with laboratory accidents or graphic descriptions of gory injuries or nasty fires should be avoided. Frightened, timid students are more likely to have accidents than the confident laboratory man who works with due regard to safety." This statement, written by J. R. Young (1) in 1971, in *The Journal of Chemical Education,* applies not only to students working in the chemical laboratory but can be extended to all scientists and technicians working with hazardous products, and in particular with chemical carcinogens.

The hazards of handling toxic or dangerous chemicals have been well documented. Besides safety notices and articles in the scientific literature, a large number of books have been dedicated to this subject, among which can be cited *Safety and Accident Prevention in Chemical Operations* (2), *Handbook of Laboratory Safety* (3), *Hazards in the Chemical Laboratory* (4),

Handbook of Reactive Chemical Hazards (5), *Safety in Working with Chemicals* (6) and *Prudent Practices for Handling Hazardous Chemicals in Laboratories* (7).

The consequences of bad laboratory practices in handling toxic or corrosive chemicals, such as burns and intoxication, can be seen over a short time, while those of exposure to carcinogenic compounds are detected only long after exposure. The handling of carcinogenic chemicals also poses more severe problems than that of toxic or corrosive chemicals, because, even though laboratory workers may be aware of these delayed effects, when they handle carcinogens daily for long periods of time, they tend to become less careful. Some studies performed among laboratory workers have demonstrated that this population is at an increased occupational risk of cancer (8–15).

Until the 1970s, only scattered information had been published concerning the handling of carcinogenic compounds, either by institutes using them (16–21) or in the scientific literature (22–23). In 1979, The International Agency for Research on Cancer (IARC) convened an international board of scientists, experts in the field of carcinogenesis, who elaborated a comprehensive document on the safe handling of chemical carcinogens (24). In the meantime, the National Institutes of Health (NIH) of the USA revised their 1975 document into a much more comprehensive one, which was published in 1980 (25). Since that time, a number of publications have appeared, either as internal guides in institutes (26–27) or in the open scientific literature 28–33, all devoted to the safe handling of carcinogenic substances. But what are carcinogenic substances, and how is the risk defined?

In the introduction to *Laboratory Use of Chemical Carcinogens* (25), the guidelines are defined as to apply to the use of chemical substances for which standards have been promulgated by the Occupational Safety and Health (OSHA) in 29 CFR 1910.1001–1045, chemical substances for which OSHA promulgates standards in the future in accordance with 29 CFR part 1990, and other chemical substances which, in the judgement of the NIH Occupational Safety and Health Committee, pose a carcinogenic risk to laboratory personnel (34–36).

In the series *IARC Monographs on the Evaluation of the Carcinogenic Risk of Chemicals to Humans* (37–73), groups of experts have reviewed data concerning chemicals, groups of chemicals and industrial processes and classified them into three main categories, as follows:

Group 1. The chemical, group of chemicals, industrial process or occupational exposure is carcinogenic to humans.

Group 2. The chemical, group of chemicals, industrial process or occupational exposure is probably carcinogenic to humans (this category is divided into higher (group A) and lower (group B) degrees of evidence).

Group 3. The chemical, group of chemicals, industrial process or occupational exposure cannot be classified as to its carcinogenicity to humans.

The *IARC Monographs* Supplement No. 4 (68) reviewed data on chemicals covered in the first 29 monographs for which there were data in humans and categorized them into the groups as follows (for all the other compounds evaluated, the degree of evidence of carcinogenicity can be found in the individual documents (69–73)).

Group 1. The Working Group concluded that the following seven industrial processes and occupational exposures and 23 chemicals and groups of chemicals are causally associated with cancer in humans[1].

Industrial processes and occupational exposures:

> Auramine manufacture
> Boot and shoe manufacture and repair (certain occupations)
> Furniture manufacture
> Isopropyl alcohol manufacture (strong-acid process)
> Nickel refining
> Rubber industry (certain occupations)
> Underground haematite mining (with exposure to radon)

Chemicals and groups of chemicals:

> 4-Aminobiphenyl
> Analgesic mixtures containing phenacetin[a]
> Arsenic and arsenic compounds[a]
> Asbestos
> Azathioprine
> Benzene
> Benzidine
> N,N-Bis(2-chloroethyl)-2-naphthylamine (Chlornaphazine)
> Bis(chloromethyl)ether and technical-grade chloromethyl methyl ether
> 1,4-Butanediol dimethanesulphonate (Myleran)
> Certain combined chemotherapy for lymphomas[a] (including MOPP[b])

---

[1] This list does not include known human carcinogens such as tobacco smoke, betel quid and alcoholic beverages, since they had not yet been covered in the *Monographs* programme.

Chlorambucil
Chromium and certain chromium compounds[a]
Conjugated oestrogens[a]
Cyclophosphamide
Diethylstilboestrol
Melphalan
Methoxsalen with ultra-violet A therapy (PUVA)
Mustard gas
2-Naphthylamine
Soots, tars and oils[a, c]
Treosulphan
Vinyl chloride

[a] The compound(s) responsible for the carcinogenic effect in humans cannot be specified.
[b] Procarbazine, nitrogen mustard, vincristine and prednisone.
[c] Mineral oils may vary in composition, particularly in relation to their content of carcinogenic polycyclic aromatic hydrocarbons.

Group 2. The following 61 chemicals, groups of chemicals or industrial processes are probably carcinogenic to humans

Group 2A

Acrylonitrile
Aflatoxins
Benzo[*a*]pyrene
Beryllium and beryllium compounds[a]
Combined oral contraceptives[a]
Diethyl sulphate
Dimethyl sulphate
Manufacture of magenta[a]
Nickel and certain nickel compounds
Nitrogen mustard
Oxymetholone
Phenacetin
Procarbazine
ortho-Toluidine

[a] The compound(s) responsible for the carcinogenic effect in humans cannot be specified.

Group 2B

Actinomycin D
Adriamycin
Amitrole
Auramine (technical grade)
Benzotrichloride
Bischloroethyl nitrosourea (BCNU)
Cadmium and cadmium compounds
Carbon tetrachloride
Chloramphenicol
1-(2-Chloroethyl)-3-cyclohexyl-1-nitrosourea
(CCNU)
Chloroform
Chlorophenols (occupational exposure to)[a]
Cisplatin
Dacarbazine
DDT
3,3'-Dichlorobenzidine
Dienoestrol
3,3'-Dimethoxybenzidine (*ortho*-Dianisidine)
Dimethylcarbamoyl chloride
1,4-Dioxane
Direct Black 38 (technical grade)
Direct Blue 6 (technical grade)
Direct Brown 95 (technical grade)
Epichlorohydrin
Ethinyloestradiol
Ethylene dibromide
Ethylene oxide
Ethylene thiourea
Formaldehyde (gas)
Hydrazine
Mestranol
Metronidazole
Norethisterone
Oestradiol-17
Oestrone
Phenazopyridine
Phenytoin
Phenoxyacetic acid herbicides (occupational exposure
to)[a]
Polychlorinated biphenyls

Progesterone
Propylthiouracil
Sequential oral contraceptives[a]
Tetrachlorodibenzo-*para*-dioxin (TCDD)
2,4,6-Trichlorophenol
Tris(aziridinyl)-*para*-benzoquinone (Triaziquone)
Tris(1-aziridinyl)phosphine sulphide (Thiotepa)
Uracil mustard

---

[a] The compound(s) responsible for the probable carcinogenic effect in humans cannot be specified.

Group 3. The remaining 64 chemicals, groups of chemicals, industrial processes and occupational exposures could not be classified as to their carcinogenicity to humans.

The fact that a monograph has been prepared on a chemical, complex mixture or occupation does not imply that the carcinogenic hazard is associated with the exposure, only that the published data have been examined. Equally, the fact that a chemical complex mixture or occupation has not yet been evaluated in the monographs does not mean that it does not represent a carcinogenic hazard.

The physical state and the physical properties of the compounds the above list vary widely; the same applies to the usage and to the quantities involved during manipulation. The two following sections attempt to pool and review comprehensively the available data (in addition to some personal views) concerning the handling and disposal of these compounds.

2 Hazards in Handling Chemical Carcinogens

2.1 Responsibilities

In all laboratories where work with chemical carcinogens is performed, the responsibilities for safe planning of experiments should be clearly defined. Since there is a great variety of administrative structures in the laboratories where such compounds are handled, however, it is difficult to provide clear guidelines in this respect. Each institute where work with chemical carcinogens is planned must set up a scale of responsibilities in the safety organization. The information in the following section, extracted from Montesano et al. (24) and NIH (25), is given as a guideline.

1) *Principal Scientific Investigator*

He has the prime responsibility, in consultation with his colleagues involved in the work and the Safety Officer, to:
1. Acquire all the information pertinent to the selection of the level of precautions to be taken;
2. Propose them;
3. Obtain approval from the Safety Committee when necessary;

9

4. Inform his employees of the danger of the compounds they will be working with, and instruct them of the procedures to be applied;
5. Ensure that all the safety procedures are applied;
6. Arrange for immediate first aid and report any accident to the Safety Committee or the supervisor.

During his or her investigation of the safety measures to be applied, the scientific officer should ask the following questions:

- What personnel would be involved in the experiment(s)?
- What is the carcinogenicity of the chemical to be used? What are its physical and chemical properties?
- How will the experiment be conducted?
- What quantity of carcinogen will be used?
- Where should the carcinogen be obtained and what is the minimum amount to be ordered compatible with the running of the experiment?
- Where will the carcinogen be stored at its arrival in the laboratory?
- Where will it be dispensed? By whom? How?
- Where should the experiment be carried out? Which minimum precautions should be applied?
- How should the room and the equipment be cleaned?
- What method should be used to assess the effectiveness of the cleaning?
- How should wastes be treated before disposal?
- How should the area where the chemical carcinogens are to be handled be protected, e.g., restriction of access, labelling, etc.?
- What protective clothing should be provided, not only to the persons working in the protected area but also to those with access to that area? Where

should they be worn? Should they be cleaned? How? Should they be disposable?

- What should the sequence of operations be in case of emergency?
- How should staff be trained and informed for the normal routine? For emergencies?

2) *The Employees*

They should be closely involved in drawing-up the details of the experiments with the principal scientific investigator. They should ensure that they understand the work and follow strictly the safety guidelines and procedure required for the task they are performing, so as not to expose themselves or their colleagues. They should report any unsafe conditions of work to their supervisor and, in case of accident, report details of the conditions that resulted, or might have resulted, in exposure.

3) *The Director*

He has the ultimate responsibility for safe operation in his department. He must therefore:

- Generate a climate in which all staff will feel personally responsible for the safety of all laboratory operations and free to report at any time any departure from good practice and possible improvements in the safety scheme;
- Provide the resources required to ensure safe operations in the laboratory;
- Ensure that all principal scientific investigators understand, accept and fulfil their duties to conduct their experiments safely;
- Ensure that the Safety Committee understands its functions and has every freedom to propose and impose improved conditions of work.

4) *The Safety Committee*

It should involve at least one safety officer and should serve as a source of information and advice to the principal scientific investigators when drawing-up their experimental protocols and developing operating procedures. It should also provide guidance to members of personnel at all levels of responsibility. It should draw any unresolved matter of safety to the attention of the director.

The Safety Committee should also visit laboratories to ensure that safety policies concerning work with chemical carcinogens are being followed.

It must investigate the reasons for any accident, report their conclusions to the director and propose action that would avoid such accidents in the future.

It should ensure that adequate training and retraining is provided to all staff, at all levels, involved with work with chemical carcinogens, including those in charge of emergency procedures, evacuation of wastes and their decontamination.

It should supervise decontamination operations when accidents have resulted in contamination of laboratory areas, and ensure that adequate methods of testing are used to ensure the effectiveness of decontamination.

2.2 Supply, Storage and Transportation of Chemical Carcinogens Outside the Laboratory (24–26, 74)

A laboratory director who wants to initiate research with chemical carcinogens must not only make sure that the work can be performed safely in his laboratory but must first localize potential suppliers of the compounds he wishes to work with. Three main sources of supply of such compounds can be envisaged — purchase from a chemical company, in-house synthesis and gifts from collaborators involved in the same field of research.

In order to reduce problems of disposal, the quantities purchased, synthethized or asked for should be as close as possible to the minimum required for the conduct of the experiments. However, it should be recognized that many chemical companies sell their products in comparatively large bulk, thus creating in-house stocks. Before placing an order for a chemical carcinogen, the scientist and/or supply officer must make sure that stock quantities of this compound are not available in-house. This will be greatly facilitated by looking into a well-maintained inventory, as described below.

Synthesis avoids the problem of transportation of chemical carcinogens from outside but requires very strict control of the laboratory operations, as discussed later in this Section. The two other means of acquiring the chemical carcinogens pose problems of transportation to the laboratory; the same problem arises when samples have to be sent to collaborating laboratories.

Before carcinogenic materials are sent, the regulations concerning their transport that are in force in the national post offices, railway, boat or airline companies should be looked at and strictly adhered to. In some cases, a company or national body may refuse to handle and transport some compounds; this is the case, for example, in respect of bis-chloromethylether, which no US airline company will accept in their freight. Even though the regulations concerning the transport of inflammable or corrosive materials are well documented (the International Air Transport Association, Dangerous Goods Regulations (75), can usefully be consulted), very few refer to known or suspected carcinogenic substances. In case of doubt, the following minimum requirements for packing of carcinogenic substances for transportation must be fulfilled (see Figure 1): The carcinogen, pure or in solution, must be placed in a primary container, leak-proof and securely sealed; this primary container is then placed in a second container, leak-proof, un-breakable, filled with enough absorbent material to completely absorb the carcinogen, if it is a liquid or in solution, and prevent any movement of the primary container, which should be able to withstand any attack from the chemical carcinogen or the solvent.

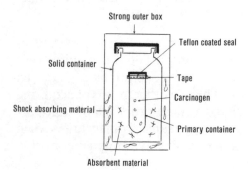

Fig. 1

The second container should then be packed in a strong outer box, large enough to accommodate it and allow the insertion all around of enough shockabsorbent material. In some cases, it will be necessary to place the second container in a thick polystyrene outer box, to which some dry ice should be added. This acts as a

14

shock-absorbing material, but may also need to be strengthened with a cardboard or wooden box.

The sender of the parcel must use the quickest means of transportation, avoiding shipment at weekends and during holiday periods, and should warn the receiver of the shipment, who can then himself (or one of his collaborators) take care of the parcel when it arrives and properly store the compounds. In addition, the sender should warn the receiver, either by letter sent before the parcel, telex or telephone, of the shipment date and route, giving details of the documents issued for the transport, such as airway bill number or number on the railway documents. If the parcel is not received within the expected time, the carrier must be notified immediately so that a search can be initiated promptly.

Immediately on receipt, stock quantities of chemical carcinogens should be handed to the requisitioner or a person designated by him and stored in places that have been chosen in advance. Although it is feasible to designate several storage places for stock quantities in the same building, it is recommended that scattering be avoided and that all pure substances be stored in one room of the building, which is fully equipped for their safe handling. Possible equipment for such a room is discussed in Section 2.6.

The compounds must be stored in cupboards or spark-free refrigerators or freezers, in trays that cannot be attacked by the chemical carcinogens.

The arrival of each new compound, or new batch of compounds, should be recorded in an inventory, which should also contain the name of the person who ordered or synthesized the compound, each vial being labelled with the name of the responsible person. Whenever a flask is emptied, the entry should be crossed off the inventory; before disposal, the vial must be decontaminated, using, for example, one of the procedures described in Section 3. Before ordering or synthesizing a compound, the scientist who requires it should check whether it is already available in the stock and enquire from colleagues responsible for the compound whether they still need it, or whether it can be made available to him. If a room has been allocated for the storage or handling of bulk quantities of carcinogens, every scientist who needs an aliquot must sample his aliquot in this room and not carry the compound in its original package out of the room; the size of the aliquot must not exceed that necessary for conducting the experiment. It can also be put into solution in this room. The aliquot itself, or its solution, properly labelled (see Section 2.3), can be carried to the laboratory where it will be used, using appropriate precautions (see Section 2.3).

Solutions can then be stored in the laboratory before use, in sparkfree freezers or refrigerators, in trays that cannot be attacked by the carcinogen or the solvent.

2.2 Identification

Proper, clear identification of a risk is the first step in its prevention. Two types of identification must be considered: that of the area where chemical carcinogens are handled, and that of all containers holding chemical carcinogens.

2.2.1 Identification of Risk Areas

As far as possible, all work with and storage of chemical carcinogens should be segregated from other work and storage places and, whenever possible, situated in laboratories or places reserved only for this purpose.

At each entrance to an area where chemical carcinogens are being handled or stored, a warning sign indicating the hazard must be displayed. This sign should be written in such a way that all persons can read and understand it. The following signs have been adopted at NIH (25) and IARC (Fig. 2).

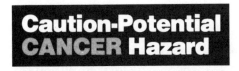

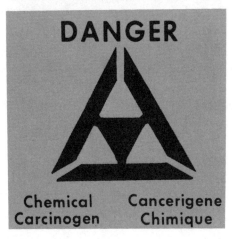

Fig. 2a and b. White letters on black background: shaded letters in red. **a.** NIH warning sign; **b.** IARC warning sign.

In any area where such signs are displayed, access should be limited to staff in charge of the experiments and to persons designated by them. To prevent incidents, visitors should always be escorted when entering laboratories where carcinogenic or potentially carcinogenic substances are handled.

Some laboratories have introduced the notion of degrees of risk and have set out two or three zones of high, moderate or low hazard (26, 74, 76). This notion of degree of danger is based on several factors, such as: the physical state of the compound, its volatility, its concentration, its biological activity, the type of experiment and the amount of carcinogenic substance handled. Other laboratories (77) distinguish between known carcinogens and presumptive chemical carcinogens (e.g., chemical mutagens or teratogens), such distinctions being reflected in the presentation of the warning sign. In addition to warning signs, one institute (26) has suggested using rubber barriers across access to areas where carcinogenic substances are being used. Such barriers and signs could be removed from areas where experiments of a temporary nature are being carried out.

When experiments involving chemical carcinogens are left in progress, the name and telephone number of the responsible officer in charge of the experiment should be left attached to the sign indicating the hazard.

2.2.2 Identification of Containers

All carcinogen containers should have labels indicating:
- whether it is pure or in solution and, in the case of solutions, the concentration and the solvent used.

This latter indication is vital in cases of spillage, as discussed in Section 3, some methods being rendered inefficient by certain solvents.

Another useful indication to add to labels is the date of preparation of the solution.

2.3 Transportation of Carcinogens Within the Laboratory

It is strongly recommended that transportation of stock quantities of chemical carcinogens be avoided within a building. To avoids this, facilities for dispensing carcinogens must be contiguous to the storage area. Aliquots of solids can be transferred in adequate vessels with the help of spatulas prior to weighing. Liquid substances can be transferred with appropriate syringes or safety pipettes to hermetically closed vessels prior to weighing, if their density is known; volumetric transfer is also an accurate way of measuring the size of an aliquot. In any case, no mouth pipetting should be performed during such transfer.

The hazard involved in the transportation of carcinogens is, therefore, reduced to that of the transportation of small aliquots. Such aliquots should nevertheless be transported to the laboratory with great care, to avoid the problem of spillage in common areas, such as corridors and lifts.

Such aliquots must be transported in unbreakable containers, which will withstand chemical attack by the carcinogen or the solvent (if a solution has already been prepared) for transportation to the laboratory. These containers should also be leak-proof and should contain some absorbing material. At IARC, stainless-steel containers resembling milk-cans have been adopted. To render them leak-proof, silicon joints have been used. The main advantage of stainless-steel is that, in case of breakage of a flask containing a chemical carcinogen inside the can, in-situ decontamination can be carried out, since this material is resistant to oxidants, acids, bases, etc.

Another transportation problem is that of waste that must be evacuated from the laboratory. Two types of wastes must be considered — small volumes of solution, moderately or highly contaminated, generated by synthesis in the laboratory or as residues; and large volumes of slightly contaminated wastes, such as animal litter resulting from biological experiments. In all cases, it is advisable to reduce to a minimum the transportation of these compounds. Several methods have now been studied for the in-situ treatment of a wide range of chemical carcinogens (see Section 3), pure or in solutions, which must be used whenever possible. Although some of these methods can be used for the treatment of large quantities of wastes, such as litter, they lead to very large volumes of heavy wastes, which are difficult to evacuate; in this case, transportation of slightly contaminated waste to a treatment area is preferable. Such wastes should be placed in plastic bags or other suitable, impermeable containers, which should be sealed and placed in solid outer containers for transportation.

All containers used for the transportation of chemical carcinogens should be identified with a warning sign.

2.4 The Problem of Spillage
(24, 76, 78, 79)

Spillage is one of the most acute problems for scientists working with chemical carcinogens. When starting an experiment with chemical carcinogens, the experimenter must foresee emergency strategies to deal with this problem.

Under the following eight headings, Meiners et al. (79) have described a strategy to reduce the problem of spillage:

1. Adequate laboratory facilities,
2. Protective equipment,
3. Appropriate laboratory techniques,
4. Planned emergency procedures,
5. Knowledge of physical and chemical properties,
6. Knowledge of decontamination procedures,
7. Appropriate analytical methodology,
8. Disposal procedures.

Adequate laboratory facilities include suitable protective clothing, extensive ventilation controls, ventilated safety cabinets or glove boxes and good surface finishes of walls, floors and ceilings. Such facilities are discussed in Section 2.5.

Protective equipment should include gloves, protective suits and respirators.

Appropriate laboratory techniques can help in limiting most spills to enclosed areas, rendering them much less hazardous and avoiding their spread.

Planned emergency procedures, including evacuation of personnel and methods of intervention, are vital in cases of spillage of a carcinogen outside an enclosed area.

Knowledge of the physical and chemical properties of a carcinogen is a necessary condition for treatment of spills.

Knowledge of decontamination procedures, their kinetics, their products, the toxicity of the products and the reversibility of the reaction should guide selection of procedures.

Appropriate analytical methodology is necessary to establish that the compound has been degraded and, in the case of volatile compounds, that it is absent from the working atmosphere.

Finally, nationally acceptable disposal procedures must be strictly followed for the elimination of decontaminated wastes.

The immediate strategy in the event of spillage might be envisaged, depending on whether the spilt carcinogen is a solid in powder form, a nonvolatile product in solution or a volatile substance, either pure or in solution.

● For a solid in powder form, the first action must be to limit its dispersion; this can be done by stopping or reducing the ventilation or movement of air.

● For a nonvolatile product in solution, the spread should be reduced immediately, by covering the area with an absorbent material.

● For volatile products, immediate evacuation and isolation of the laboratory should be the first step.

In all cases, all personnel working in the vicinity of a spill should be alerted, and safety personnel notified of the nature of the spill. Whenever possible, in-situ decontamination of the spill area must be performed, thereby limiting handling of the carcinogen or its solutions, which might penetrate protective clothing or respirators (see Section 3.2).

Immediately after decontamination and clean-up, personnel should discard the protective clothing and wash with only soap and water.

2.5 Protection of Staff (24—26, 78)

The first step in protecting staff is prevention, which entails the provision of full information about the purpose and dangers of the experiments they are carrying out and adequate training concerning good personnel practices and good experimental practices. Adequate laboratory installations and protective clothing are an aid to this protection.

2.5.1 Personnel Practices

In laboratories where chemical carcinogens are used or stored, no eating, drinking, smoking, chewing of gum or tobacco, cosmetic or make-up application should be allowed. Storage of food or beverages or of containers or utensils that might be used with them should be prohibited. Laboratory glassware or utensils should never be used for drinking or eating purposes.

Pipetting must always be performed using mechanical systems. Oral pipetting of known or suspected chemical carcinogens, their solutions, or of toxic compounds, should not, under any circumstances be allowed.

During all operations in which chemical carcinogens are involved, all personnel should wear protective clothing (see Section 2.5 (3)), which they must remove following completion of the experiments and, in any case, when they leave the laboratory. Such protective clothing should include shoes in all areas where laboratory animals treated with chemical carcinogens are handled. When leaving the laboratory, personnel should also wash their hands and, if possible and where appropriate, as in the case of staff working with laboratory animals, shower.

Eye protection devices, appropriate to the type of work performed, should be used in the laboratory work area.

With regard to the employment of pregnant women in laboratories where chemical carcinogens are handled, medical and legal advice should be sought, and each institution should adopt an appropriate policy.

2.5.2 Experimental Practices

All operations in which volatile carcinogens are handled (chemical or biochemical, microbiological and cell-culture experiments (80) as well as animal treatment) or in which a chemical carcinogen may be rendered volatile by some physical or chemical means (synthesis, purification by distillation or sublimation, some analytical procedures such as injection into a gas chromatograph (81), gas chromatographic analysis using non-destructive detectors, melting-point determination) must be performed under wellventilated hoods and, in some cases, by personnel wearing respirators. During in-vitro carcinogenicity tests involving N-nitrosodimethylamine, Huberman et al. (82) demonstrated that up to 25% of the amount of carcinogen added to culture medium in petri dishes in an incubator was lost, and its presence could be demonstrated in dishes to which it had not been added. The same applies to all operations that may result in the generation of aerosols, such as the opening of closed vessels, transfer operations, the preparation of feed mixtures (83), blending, open-vessel centrifugation, injection or intubation of chemical carcinogens into experimental animals, and scraping of thin-layer chromatography plates (84).

Nonvolatile carcinogens can be sampled outside a hood. When working with some very light powders, it is essential that there be very low or no air draft, which would facilitate dispersion; for such compounds, it is advisable to sample them outside of a well ventilated-hood. If available, a glove box can be used instead. Another alternative is to dissolve the carcinogen in a suitable solvent, upon arrival at the laboratory, thus reducing the handling problem to that of a solution.

Some compounds behave like electrostatic powders — e. g., some mycotoxins, polycyclic aromatic hydro-carbons. In handling these in powder form, under no circumstances should synthetic clothing (latex or vinyl gloves, synthetic face masks) be worn, which would facilitate dispersion. To reduce the problem of han-dling such compounds, they can be put into solution on arrival, so that only an aliquot of a solution of a nonvolatile carcinogen need be taken.

All work surfaces on which chemical carcinogens are used should be protected. When carcinogens are used in powder form, a paper cloth or dry absorbent plastic-backed paper may be used. When carcinogens are used in liquid form or in solutions, trays covered with one of the previously described absorbing materials must be used. Such trays should be of a material that cannot be attacked by either the carcinogen or the solvent.

When analytical instruments, e. g., analytical balances, are used in the course of manipulation of chemical carcinogens, the sample should be placed in tightly stoppered tubes or vials, so as to avoid contamination. If, by accident, analytical instruments become contaminated, they should not be used until they have been thoroughly decontaminated (see Section 3).

Use of respirators equipped with filter cartridges for removal of particulate or organic vapour cartridges or a combination of both should be a normal laboratory habit for all persons, including maintenance and emergency personnel, entering areas that have been contaminated. These should also be used in exceptional cases for people working with very volatile compounds or aerosols in front of hoods where turbulence may create a back draft of vapours or aerosols.

In order to avoid a build-up of contamination, which could occur during continuous conduct of experiments, regular monitoring of surfaces such as floors, benches, walls, interiors of hoods and air ducts, and of the atmosphere, must be performed. Simple and sensitive methods for sampling and analysis should be used for monitoring contamination. Some of these are described or referenced in *IARC Scientific Publications* Nos. 18, 22, 29, 40, 45 and 46 (85–90). Such a monitoring programme must also be extended to the testing of surfaces after decontamination of a spill.

Whenever an area (bench, floor or entire room) has been contaminated, it must be cleaned immediately using appropriate methods (see Section 3.2), when available. Such cleaning must be performed by laboratory personnel or by an emergency team who are properly trained, and should not be left to the usual house-cleaning staff. When no contamination has occurred, the floor may be cleaned by the usual house-cleaning staff; but working surfaces should always be cleaned by laboratory personnel. Laboratories must be cleaned in such a way as to avoid producing aerosols or dispersing dust. Wet cleaning and the use of highly-efficient vacuum cleaners, fitted with particulate filters, are to be recommended.

Glassware and laboratory utensils should be decontaminated completely by laboratory personnel before being sent for washing. Decontamination may be effected by appropriate methodologies (see Section 3), when available, or by rinsing several times with adequate volumes of a suitable solvent. In some cases, four to five rinses have been found to be sufficient to achieve good decontamination.

Animal rooms are bound to be contaminated (91–94). Means for minimizing such contamination should include:
- Administration of volatile carcinogens preferably by injection of solutions; gavage occasions aerosol formation, mixing with food or drink occasions evaporation or aerosol formations and both operations must be performed under a well ventilated-hood;
- Placing animals under a hood whenever experiments are performed in which a chemical carcinogen may be exhaled;
- Mixing of carcinogens with food in sealed mixers under a hood;
- Placing animals treated with contaminated diet or drink or by skin painting in cages with solid bottoms and sides, with a filter top (except when volatile carcinogens are used);

- Decontaminating cages that have been used to house animals treated with chemical carcinogens;
- Installing cage-cleaning facilities in the area where the animals are being treated to avoid moving contaminated cages to other areas.

Animal houses must be cleaned by the animal caretakers themselves, who should be fully trained to deal with contamination and be protected against all its aspects. Such cleaning, as described above, should be performed in such a way as to avoid production of aerosols and diffusion of dust. Therefore, only wet cleaning is recommended, since the exhaust of a vacuumcleaner will redisperse what animals have diffused, which will settle on trays, walls, outside cages, etc. Neither dry sweeping nor dry mopping, which might generate aerosols, should be used.

Removal of filters from exhausts, hoods or air conditioning units should be performed in such a way that the person doing it is at no time in contact with the filter or the filter housing (see Section 2.5 (4)).

2.5.3 Laboratory Installations

In order to avoid accumulation of carcinogens in angles between floors and walls or their penetration in the case of spillage, and to facilitate cleaning, rooms in which carcinogens are handled should not have absorbent materials on the floor or walls, and tiling should be avoided. Whenever possible, floors and walls should be covered with impermeable material, which should be continuous from the floor to the wall, without edges, and which, if wetted accidentally, should be of a type that will not become dangerously slippery.

At least in high-risk areas (where pure chemical carcinogenic substances are handled), the ceiling must be of one piece, impermeable and fixed to the walls, so that the only connections between the whole room, and neighbouring laboratories or corridors are the door, the ventilation system and the hood exhaust.

Whenever a ventilation system is available in the laboratories, its exhaust should contain filters; all exhaust air from high risk zones must be filtered. The filter should comprise at least a fibre filter for dust and a charcoal filter for vapours. Breakthrough volumes of some carcinogens and solvents through charcoal have been studied by Sansone and Jonas (95).

The atmospheric pressure in areas in which chemical carcinogens are handled should always be negative with regard to that of neighbouring laboratories and corridors. In their guide to safe handling of non-radioactive chemical carcinogens in laboratories, Le Neveu et al. (26) distinguish three levels of risk in the handling of chemical carcinogens and propose that, in the high-hazard areas, there should be a minimum of eight volumes of air changes per hour, and that with medium-hazard areas, a pressure differential of 5–10 mm of water be maintained. Medium-hazard areas should have a lower pressure than low-hazard areas, which should have a lower pressure than offices or corridors. The pressure differential between medium-risk areas and offices or corridors should be maintained at 15–45 mm of water. In this way, if there is contamination, it can only enter a higher-risk zone.

Hoods should be installed in all areas where chemical carcinogens are handled and should be equipped with efficient filters, as described above for the ventilation systems. Several suggestions, ranging from

0.5–1 m/s, have been made concerning the face velocity of air. The most informative report is that of Le Neveu et al. (26), who suggest that 0.75 m/s, with a sash opening of 460 mm, be maintained. The efficiency of hoods should be checked periodically — quarterly seems a good average time. They should work permanently, and should be used as part or all of the room exhaust and no shut-off switch should be available in the room. An alarm should be installed in cases of misfunctioning.

When installed, glove boxes must be kept under a negative pressure of 15–45 mm of water with respect to the space in which they are located. However, personnel should be made aware of the problems of gloves (see Section 2.5 (4)).

It is recommended that benches be made of impermeable material, and that trays be available in a material that cannot be attacked by carcinogens or solvents. Stainless-steel trays are preferable, since they can also resist acids and strong oxidants, which might be necessary for their decontamination (see Section 3). Absorbent material with a plastic undercoating must be provided for placing on benches and in trays.

Eye-wash facilities and safety showers must be installed in every laboratory where chemical carcinogens are used.

2.5.4 Protective Clothing and Equipment

Protective clothing and equipment should be the last defense against contamination by chemical carcinogens. However, they should always be worn when dealing with these compounds.

No protective clothing should be worn outside laboratory areas. Disposable protective clothing should be discarded in a safe manner, and reusable protective clothing, if not contaminated, can be washed. After contamination, reusable protective clothing should not be sent to the laundry before being decontaminated. If no method of decontamination is available, the clothing must be discarded in a safe manner.

The minimal protective clothing to be worn in a chemical or biochemical laboratory is a fully fastened, long laboratory coat. As described by Barbeito (78), this could be replaced by a fully buttoned laboratory coat, wrap-around smock, solid front gown, one-piece laboratory suit, heavy-duty overall or two-piece laboratory suit. For personnel working with laboratory animals, completely closed jump-suits are preferable; in addition, such staff should be provided with shoes or boots, head cover and gloves. Suitable respiratory protection may also be used to avoid breathing in the dust and aerosols generated by animals; in this case, face masks are preferable to respirators, which should not be used for routine operations but only under exceptional conditions.

Cotton face masks should be provided to persons working with electrostatic powders in chemical laboratories. In this case, also, respirators should be used only under exceptional conditions and not in a routine manner.

A complete set of clothing should be put at the disposal of security or laboratory staff in charge of emergency decontamination. This should include a respirator equipped with filter cartridges for particulate removal or appropriate organic vapour cartridges or a combination of both, a self-contained breathing apparatus, thick rubber boots, thick rubber gloves and a plastic disposable suit. Training will be provided for the use of the self-contained breathing apparatus.

There remains the problem of gloves. In areas where pure chemical carcinogens are handled, disposable cotton gloves should be provided and are preferable to latex or vinyl gloves for handling electrostatic powders, such as aflatoxins and polycyclic aromatic hydrocarbons. Rubber, latex or vinyl gloves can be used for all other operations with pure compounds or their solutions. However, it must be remembered that such gloves do not provide full protection, not only in the case of pure liquid carcinogens, which when they are in contact with gloves diffuse through the latex (95–100), but also for solid compounds in solutions (101–102), the diffusion in this case being favourized by the action of some solvents on the glove material (103). Walker et al. (98) proposed using two pairs of gloves separated by a layer of barrier cream or talcum powder when handling compounds like volatile nitrosamines, a precaution which can be extended to any other situation. When handling aflatoxins in chloroform, Castegnaro et al. (102) proposed the use of two pairs of gloves to reduce the transfer of the solution. Nevertheless, whenever contamination of gloves occurs, they should be removed as quickly as possible, decontaminated and discarded.

In glove boxes, gloves are much more difficult to change and their use might result in a permanently contaminated zone (which should be avoided as far as possible) or dispersal of the compound through the glove into the room, thereby contaminating it. In all cases, when using a glove box, laboratory personnel should wear at least one pair of disposable gloves dusted with talcum powder. In my view, efficient hoods are preferable to glove boxes.

2.6 Some Considerations for Building a Room in which Pure Carcinogenic Substances can be Handled

The above sections indicate some guidelines for the minimum requirements of a room in which undiluted chemical carcinogens will be handled. These are described in detail here.

2.6.1 The Room Itself

It must be built in such a way that there is no possibility of any contamination escaping into corridors or other rooms in the building or outside the building. All exhaust systems, i.e., air-conditioning ducts, hoods and drains, should be equipped with adequate trapping systems, which can be changed by maintenance personnel without manual contact. The room should have a minimum of eight air changes per hour and a minimum of 5 mm of water pressure differential with other laboratory areas to which they are linked and/or 10–20 mm of water pressure differential with offices or corridors.

The floor should not be made of tiles (to avoid joints where contamination might accumulate) but should be covered with a monolithic, impermeable material, which should be continuous from the floor to the walls, without edges.

An antechamber should be built at the entrance to the room, where disposable protective equipment, such as laboratory coats, cotton, latex or vinyl gloves, cotton face masks, respirators and safety spectacles, are available and where there is a complete set of clothing for personnel in charge of emergency decontamination. The antechamber should have glass windows giving onto the room and should be maintained at a minimum of 5 mm of water positive pressure differential with respect to the room.

The entrance to the room should be clearly labelled to indicate the hazard.

2.6.2 Equipment of the Room

Storage facilities should be installed for chemical carcinogens, which could include cupboards and spark-free freezers and/or refrigerators equipped with trays that cannot be attacked by carcinogens.

An inventory of the names and storage area of all carcinogens, and the names of the scientists responsible for them, should be affixed to the storage places.

Hoods should be installed with a face velocity of 0.5 to 0.75 m/s, with a sash opening of about 40 cm. As described above, the hood exhaust should be equipped with filters and an alarm system, in case of malfunction, and should be built to function permanently. The working surface might be in the form of a cuvette, and in any case should be made of an impermeable material.

The surfaces of benches should be covered with an impermeable material that cannot be attacked by carcinogens or by the solvents that might be used to dilute them. Trays that can resist attack by carcinogens, and solvents and absorbent material for benches and trays, should be placed on the benches, with scissors and adhesive tape to cut and fix the absorbing material.

Unbreakable, leak-proof containers that can withstand chemical attack by carcinogens or solvents should be available for transportation of carcinogens. They should be of different sizes to accommodate different types of glassware and should contain absorbent material that can also act as a shock-absorber.

Trays and transportation containers can be made of stainless-steel or enamel; both should be resistant to carcinogens, solvents and any material should be installed in the room as close as possible to the hoods and the bench.

Alarm and emergency systems should be installed. All freezers should be equipped with a noise alarm system, which can be heard in other sections of the building. An emergency system that will stop all ventilation in case of breakage of containers of carcinogens in a light powder form would be useful to reduce dissemination of carcinogens into the room. Another emergency system, to increase the ventilation rate, could also be usefully installed to clear the atmosphere rapidly in case of breakage of a container of a volatile chemical carcinogen.

The above description is intended only as a guideline for the minimum requirements for the installation of a high-risk area where pure chemical carcinogens can be stored and handled safely, and additional equipment could be installed.

3 Methods for Disposal of Chemical Carcinogens and Spillage Treatment

3.1 General Considerations on Methods of Treatment and on the Type of Waste or Spillage to be Treated

"Good laboratory waste management begins with preventive measures, that is, identification of steps that can be taken to reduce the volume of chemicals that enter the waste disposal process and to prevent unusual, difficult disposal problems." In this statement, Joyce (104) summarizes the first step to be taken when setting up an experiment to approach sensibly a disposal problem. Although written for the more general problem of laboratory chemicals, it applies strictly to that of chemical carcinogens.

While a number of books general guidelines and procedures for disposing of chemical waste and handling spillage problems (2, 105–109), none deals specifically with carcinogenic substances. Only a few references can be found in the *Laboratory Waste Disposal Manual* (107). In their review of the situation, Montesano et al. (24) recommended that "Research into methods for the destruction and disposal of chemical carcinogens is urgently needed".

Carcinogenic substances should never be disposed of through drains or by evaporation into the atmosphere, nor should they be buried since they might be released later.

Carcinogenic substances should be treated in such a way that:

- the degradation products are non-toxic and non-carcinogenic;
- the procedures involved for treatment and disposal do not result in exposure to these substances of personnel in charge of the work; and
- the procedures involved for treatment and disposal do not result in contamination of equipment or space.

Two main categories of waste can be envisaged:
- large volumes of lightly contaminated wastes, such as bedding from animal experiments, carcasses and disposable protective clothing not obviously contaminated; and
- small volumes of more highly contaminated wastes, such as residues of chemical synthesis and of solutions used in biochemical or biological laboratories.

For the first category of waste, incineration may be the only feasible method of degrading carcinogenic substances and those of their metabolites that might be harmful. However, there is a large range of incinerators, the performance of which differs widely; and, for comparable equipment, the efficiency of the incineration process differs in a number of parameters, such as retention time of the compounds, feed rate and air supply of the furnaces. Few studies have been done on the efficiency of degradation of chemical carcinogens and the resulting products. Some work conducted at the National Center for Toxicological Research, Food and Drug Administration, Jefferson, AR 72079,

USA has shown that 2-acetylaminofluorene may be destroyed by incineration at 1500 °F (737 °C), measured in the secondary chamber of the incinerator with a minimum residence time of 2 sec (cited by Barbeito (78)). In an investigation of incineration conditions, the thermal decomposition of some polycyclic aromatic hydrocarbons and some halogenated analogues were studies (110). Even at temperatures as high as 725 °C, 10–19% of naphthalene compounds were still present, and 0.21% of benzo[e]pyrene. Rappe (111) has demonstrated that chlorinated dioxins are stable at temperatures up to 800 °C and that at temperatures of 300–500 °C, these compounds are formed from pre-dioxins and 2,4,5-trichlorophenol. Wilkinson and Rogers (112) evaluated five incinerators for their capacity to degrade a standard charge of 18 noncarcinogenic compounds by monitoring the exhaust for both the original charge and NO_x, SO_x, C_xH_x, HCl, CO and CO_2. Three of the units gave satisfactory results, but the authors concluded that before they were used to incinerate carcinogens, mutagens, teratogens, further research was required. A number of such studies would be necessary, not only to assess the efficiency of incineration to degrade chemical carcinogens, but also to determine whether the residues produced either in the gas stream or in aqueous effluents are noncarcinogenic.

The efficiency of incineration systems might be improved by equipping the chimney with low temperature catalytic systems, which have been demonstrated to degrade efficiently some polycyclic aromatic hydrocarbons and aflatoxins (113).

The use of incineration generates the problem of transportation of the contaminated wastes to the incinerator. In the section "Requirements for pathological incinerators", Rosenhaft (114) proposes that "Procedures for transporting pathological waste must be carefully designed so that the possibility of endangering the health of waste handlers or others that might come into contact with it are eliminated. For example, large dead animals (dogs, cats, non-human primates) may be placed in plastic-lined paper bags or in red plastic sacks and then in specially designed containers with tops tied or stapled to confine the contents completely. Waste should be transported to incinerators in licenced trucks or vans." Such procedures, although originally designed for pathological wastes can also be applied to large quantities of lightly contaminated biological wastes. However, whenever possible, automatization should be applied, to avoid handling the wastes; for example, litter can be aspirated into a large closed tank, from which it can be delivered automatically to the incinerator.

It should also be recognized that only a few laboratories have a hazardous waste incinerator, because this technique is very expensive to run. More economical alternatives to this technique should be looked at, and biodegradation might merit some attention for large volumes of lightly contaminated wastes.

Moreover, incineration does not offer a solution to the problem of spillage and is not adapted to the treatment of the second category of wastes as defined above. Since alternative techniques that would be applicable to both of these fields are necessary, the IARC and the Division of Safety of the NIH undertook a programme for the evaluation of chemical methods of decontamination of chemical carcinogens (115). At the time of their evaluation of the bibliography on this subject, Montesano et al. (24) stressed the lack of publications and that, as will be outlined later, most of the methods described in the literature were incompletely studied, and that their efficiency had been evaluated only by monitoring the disappearance of parent compounds.

At a 1979 meeting of IARC and NIH (116), the participants decided that the minimum criteria to validate a method of degradation of chemical carcinogens were as follows:

- The method should afford efficient degradation of the compounds, as detecteded by conventional, sensitive analytical techniques.
- The residues produced should be tested in the Ames mutation assay (117–118), using several strains of *Salmonela typhimurium,* with and without metabolic activation, and should not be mutagenic. When adopting this decision, it was recognized that long-term testing would provide better assurance of the absence of adverse biological effects of the residues, but that this would slow down drastically research in this field, where there is an urgent requirement for data.
- The method should be applicable in all laboratories, and should give comparable results. To meet this requirement, all the methods should be drafted in an ISO format, subjected to collaborative study and the results reviewed by the group of scientists that took part in these studies, with the object of accepting, modifying or discarding the methods.

Using this approach, methods were established for the degradation of selected compounds in the following seven classes of chemical carcinogens: aflatoxins, nitrosamines, nitrosamides, polycyclic aromatic hydrocarbons, hydrazines, haloethers and aromatic amines. A first study was also set up to investigate methods of degradation of some antineoplastic agents, a group of carcinogenic substances widely used in hospitals.

During this investigation, several attempts were made to use mixtures of chromic/sulfuric acid for the degradation of carcinogenic substances. The results, successful and unsuccessful, are presented in the following sections, but the method was not considered acceptable because of the risk of handling such reagents (119–120) and because of the regulations in force in several countries, which prohibit discharge of chromate solutions into sewage.

3.2 Methods for Chemical Treatment of Individual Carcinogens

3.2.1 Aflatoxins

Aflatoxins are natural contaminants of food and feed, and the ease of with which they develop causes great economic problems. This is probably why the establishment of methods for their destruction has received greater attention (121–125) than that of other carcinogens. Methods have been proposed for the treatment of laboratory wastes and spillage of aflatoxins by reaction with sodium hypochlorite, alkaline agents and oxidizing agents. These methods were reinvestigated using the above-mentioned criteria.

(i) *Method using treatment with sodium hypochlorite:* this method was shown to achieve efficient degradation of aflatoxins, however; when a chloroform extract of degradation mixtures from aflatoxin B_1 was tested for mutagenic activity, a strong effect was observed in *S. typhimurium* TA100, with and without metabolic activation. This activity was later assigned

Table 1. Decontamination of wastes onctaining aflatoxins

Waste category	Recommended destruction method no. (in order of preference)[a]
Stock quantities	1, 4
Spills	1
Aqueous solutions	1, 4
Nonaqueous solutions	1, 4
Petri dish contents	1
Equipment	1
Animal carcasses	3
Animal litter	2
Work-surface decontamination	1
Space decontamination	1
Clothing	1
Filtration systems	1

[a] Method 1: Destruction of aflatoxins in laboratory wastes using sodium hypochlorite;
Method 2: Destruction of aflatoxins in animal feed and litter using ammoniation;
Method 3: Degradation of aflatoxins in carcasses;
Method 4: Destruction of aflatoxins in laboratory wastes by potassium permanganate.

to 2,3-dichloroaflatoxin B_1 (129), a potent carcinogen and mutagen (130), which is unstable in solutions containing 5% acetone. A second step in the decontamination procedure was therefore introduced in which 5% acetone was added, after dilution of the hypochlorite strength to $1–1.5\%$ to avoid a strong haloform reaction.

Thus modified, the method was adopted after collaborative study for treatment of the wastes presented in Table 1 (131).

(ii) *Methods using treatment with an alkaline reagent:* Treatment of aflatoxins with an alkaline reagent at room temperature leads to opening of the lactone ring (132), and several methods using sodium hydroxide, sodium carbonate, ammonia or amines have been proposed in the literature. Treatment with sodium hydroxide or sodium carbonate achieved efficient disappearance of aflatoxins, as verified by thin-layer chromatographic analysis of a chloroform extract; however, after neutralization of the medium, the ring closes, and some re-formation of aflatoxins was observed in both cases. These two methods were therefore rejected.

Re-formation of the lactone ring can be avoided by decarboxylation at high temperature of the intermediate formed during opening by the alkaline reagent. A method using autoclaving in the presence of ammonia was therefore proposed and adopted after trial in the collaborative study. This method could be applied for treatment of animal litter (see Table 1).

(iii) *Methods using treatment with oxidizing agent:* Two methods, one involving potassium permanganate/sulfuric acid and the other a mixture of chromic and sulfuric acids, were subjected to collaborative study. Both were found satisfactory, but the method involving chromic/sulfuric acid was rejected because of the potential danger of the reagents. The field of application of the other oxidation method is presented in Table 1.

3.2.2 N-Nitrosamines

Although *N*-nitrosamines are receiving increasing attention, in contrast to aflatoxins, little effort has been made to develop methods for their degradation. Three related publications in the literature reported use reduction (133), denitrosation by acid halides (134) and oxidation (135). Eights methods in all were evaluated for their efficiency to degrade *N*-nitrosamines; six were subjected to collaborative study, and five were finally recommended by the collaborating group.

(1) *Methods using reduction:* In 1974, Gangolli et al. (133) proposed decontamination of liquid wastes contaminated by *N*-nitrosamines by reduction with aluminium foil in sodium hydroxide solution; however, this method was later found to produce hydrazines (136–137), another class of carcinogenic substances, thus exchanging one risk for another. An improvement to the method was suggested in 1981 by Lunn et al. (138–139) who used a nickel-aluminium alloy instead of aluminium. With this method, *N*-nitrosamines were first reduced to hydrazines and amines, depending on the substituents of the amino nitrogen, and then the hydrazines formed were cleaved to amines by the activated nickel powder, which had adsorbed oxygen. The efficiency of this method was confirmed during collaborative testing. Its field of application is presented in Table 2 (140). Another reduction method, using cuprous chloride, was found during the collaborative study to give non-reproducible results and was therefore rejected.

(ii) *Methods using oxidation of N-nitrosamines:* Oxidation of *N*-nitrosamines by a mixture of chromic/sulfuric acid was suggested as a decontamination technique by Ehrenberg and Wachtmeister (135) in 1979. When reinvestigated (141), this method was found to be unsatisfactory because, even when an undiluted oxidizing mixture was used, up to four days were necessary to achieve better than 99% degradation of *N*-nitrosodimethylamine; moreover, when a 50% diluted oxidizing mixture was used, up to 88% of each

Table 2. Decontamination of wastes containing
N-nitrosamines

A. Decontamination of media

Waste category	Recommended destruction method no. (in order of preference)[a]
Undiluted N-nitrosamine	1, 5, 2, 4
Spills of aqueous solutions	2
Spills of dichloromethane or ethanol solutions	1
Aqueous solutions	5, 2, 1, 4
Solutions in dichloromethane	1, 5, 4
Solutions in ethanol	5, 1
Solutions in olive oil	5
Content of petri dishes	5, 1

B. Decontamination of glassware

Type of contaminant	Recommended decontamination method[a]			
	Method 3			Method 1
	Dichloromethane	Methanol	Water	
Undiluted N-nitrosamines				×
Aqueous solutions			×	×
Alcoholic solutions	×	×	×	×
Oily solutions				×
Dichloromethane	×			×

[a] Method 1: Destruction of N-nitrosamines in laboratory wastes using denitrosation with hydrobromic acid;

Method 2: Destruction of N-nitrosamines in laboratory wastes using potassium permanganate;

Method 3: Decontamination of N-nitrosamine contaminated glassware;

Method 4: Decontamination of laboratory wastes using triethyloxonium salts;

Method 5: Destruction of N-nitrosamines in laboratory wastes using nickel-aluminium alloy in potassium hydroxide solution.

of the seven N-nitrosamines tested was found in the degradation mixture. For these reasons and that presented in Section 3.1, the method was not subject to collaborative testing.

Several laboratories suggested oxidation of N-nitrosamines with hypochlorite solutions. When testing the method with a 12.4% w/w (48° Cl) solution of sodium hypochlorite, more than 80% of each of the seven N-nitrosamines tested was present in the reaction mixture after 24 hours.

Oxidation of N-nitrosamines by potassium permanganate/sulfuric acid, although it produces N-nitramines, another class of chemical carcinogens, at an intermediate stage, produced nonmutagenic residues and was accepted after collaborative study (see Table 2 for fields of application).

(iii) *Methods using denitrosation:* Nitroso groups can be cleaved from N-nitrosamines by a mixture of hydrobromic acid in glacial acetic acid (142–143). By studying the kinetics of denitrosation of several N-nitrosamines, it was found that most undergo complete reaction in less than 15 min, except N-nitrosopyrrolidine for which 90 min were necessary to achieve 99.9% degradation (140). Alcohol was shown to retard denitrosation and water and dimethyl sulfoxide to inhibit the reaction strongly. Table 2 presents the fields of application of this method, which was agreed after satisfactory results in a collaborative study.

(iv) *Decontamination of glassware:* The previous method could be used to decontaminate glassware decontamination, but, as an alternative, five successive rinses with a suitable solvent were found to be satisfactory (see Table 2).

(v) *Method using treatment of N-nitrosamine: triethyl-oxonium tetrafluoroborate salts* (144): According to Hünig (14), *N*-nitrosamines in solution in dichloroethane form stable salts with triethyloxonium tetrafluoroborate salts, which, when treated with a strong base, evolve nitrogen. Such salts can also be formed quantitatively in dichloromethane solution and the solvent removed without reformation of the *N*-nitrosamine (145). No mutagenic activity was detected in *S. typhimurium* TA98 or TA100, with or without metabolic activation, after treatment of the *N*-nitrosamine salts with a strong base. This technique was, therefore, proposed as a possible decontamination method and accepted after collaborative testing (see Table 2 for possible fields of application).

3.2.3 N-Nitrosamides

If little had been done to evaluate techniques for the degradation of *N*-nitrosamines, even less had been done with regard to *N*-nitrosamides. Stability studies on these compounds were undertaken only in relation to biological experiments, and none were directed to studying the biological effects of the degradation products. Two reviews (146–147) mention possible reactions that might be used to degrade *N*-nitrosamides, including treatment with aqueous acid or alkaline solutions, action of hydrobromic acid, and photochemical and thermal treatments.

Treatments in the presence of alkaline reagents may evolve diazoalkanes, which are toxic gases and at least one of which (diazomethane) induces tumours in mice and rats. These methods, which were highly recommended for use with *N*-nitrosamines, could not therefore be used for degradation of *N*-nitrosamides.

Four methods were proposed and accepted with some limitations after collaborative study testing (148–149). They comprise denitrosation with a strong hydrogen halide and oxidation reactions.

(i) *Methods using denitrosation with a strong hydrogen halide:* N-nitrosamides are dissociated to nitrous acid and amides by treatment with 6 mol/L hydrochloric acid. This reaction served as a basis for two methods proposed by Sansone and Lunn (149) for degradation of N-methylnitrosourea, N-ethylnitrosourea, N-methylnitrosourethane, N-ethylnitrosourethane, N-methyl-N'-nitro-N-nitrosoguanidine and N-ethyl-N'-nitro-N-nitrosoguanidine. After this first denitrosation step, a second stage was added to avoid re-formation of N-nitrosamides, which involved the addition, in the first method, of sulfamic acid as a nitrite trapping agent, and in the second method, of iron filings, to achieve nitrite reduction. Some mutagenic activity in *S. typhimurium* TA1530, TA1535 and TA100, was seen after treatment of N-ethylnitrosourethane with the first method, and after treatment of N-ethylnitrourethane and N-methyl- and N-ethyl-N'-nitro-N-nitrosoguanidine and treatment of all N-nitrosamides in the presence of acetone by the second method. With these exceptions, both methods were accepted after collaborative testing (see Table 3 for specific fields of application).

A third denitrosation method involved use, as for N-nitrosamines, of the action of hydrobromic acid in glacial acetic acid. The reaction was very fast – less than 10 min were required to achieve better than 99.9% degradation – but re-formation was observed and it was necessary to remove the nitrosylbromide. After investigation of several possible chemical reagents, flushing out with nitrogen was found to be the most

Table 3. Decontamination of wastes containing N-nitrosamides

Waste category	Recommended destruction method no. (in order of preference)[a]
Undiluted N-nitrosamide	1, 4, 2, 3
Solutions in methanol	1, 3, 4, 2
Solutions in ethanol	1, 3, 4, 2
Solutions in dimethyl sulfoxide	1, 4, 2
Solutions in volatile organic solvents, including dichloromethane and ethyl acetate	4, 3
Solutions in acetone	1, 4, 3
Solutions in water	1, 3, 2
Spills of aqueous solutions	3
Spills of pure compound	4
Spills of solutions in organic solvents, excluding dimethyl sulfoxide	4
Contents of petri dishes	4
Solid wastes	4
Glassware	3, 4

[a] All methods are not applicable to all N-nitrosamides; see related sections in the text.

Method 1: Destruction of N-nitrosamides in laboratory wastes using sulfamic acid in hydrochloric acid solution;

Method 2: Destruction of N-nitrosamides in laboratory wastes using iron filings in hydrochloric acid solution;

Method 3: Destruction of N-nitrosamides in laboratory wastes using potassium permanganate in sulfuric acid;

Method 4: Destruction of N-nitrosamides in laboratory wastes using hydrobromic acid.

satisfactory system (148). As with N-nitrosamines, ethanol strongly retards the denitrosation reactions, and water and dimethyl sulfoxide inhibit them. Except with reaction mixtures from N-methylnitrosourea, no mutagenic activity was detected, and, after satisfactory collaborative testing, the method was adopted (149) (see Table 3 for fields of application).

(ii) *Method using oxidation with potassium permanganate/sulfuric acid:* Since oxidation by potassium permanganate/sulfuric acid proved to be very efficient for the degradation of N-nitrosamines, it was also tested for the treatment of N-nitrosamides. Less than 5 min were found to be sufficient to achieve complete disappearance of the compounds, but highly mutagenic residues were formed (148). The mutagenicity was completely suppressed by increasing the amount of oxidant and allowing eight hours of reaction. After reproducible results were obtained during the collaborative study, the method was accepted for the fields of application presented in Table 3 (149).

3.2.4 Polycyclic Aromatic Hydrocarbons

Much interest has been directed for many years to polycyclic aromatic hydrocarbons (PAH), and some studies were found in the literature of methods for the degradation of these compounds; however, the majority dealt with benzo[a]pyrene and with the decontamination of aqueous media (150–157). Only two publications addressed the problem of decontamination of laboratory wastes and of working areas (135, 158), both involving use of dichromate solutions.

Since PAH are highly susceptible to oxidation (159), several oxidation techniques were tested for efficiency of degradation, including treatment with chromic/sulfuric acid, potassium permanganate under neutral and acidic conditions and sodium hypochlorite. Two other possible destruction methods were tested, involving treatment with undiluted sulfuric acid (as suggested by Dr. G. Grimmer, personal communication) and reduction with nickel-aluminium alloy under alkaline conditions. The latter method produced non-reproducible data and was discarded.

(i) *Methods using oxidation:* Four oxidation methods were tested for the degradation of benz[a]anthracene, 7,12-dimethylbenzo[a]anthracene, benzo[a]pyrene, dibenzo[a,h]anthracene, 7-bromomethylbenz[a]anthracene and 3-methylcholanthene.

Treatment with sodium hypochlorite was not efficient in degrading these PAH, and evaluation of this method was discontinued.

Oxidation with potassium dichromate/sulfuric acid achieved more than 99% destruction of all the PAH tested, and nonmutagenic residues were obtained. Despite the good reproducibility obtained during the collaborative study, the method was discarded for the reasons outlined in Section 3.1.

Treatment with two other oxidizing mixtures, an aqueous saturated solution of potassium permanganate and 0.3 mol/L potassium permanganate in 3 mol/L sulfuric acid, was also evaluated. Both oxidants were tested with the PAH in the solid state and in solution in a technical-grade aprotic solvent, which would favour dissolution of the PAH in the reaction medium. Acetone, dimethylformamide and dimethylsulfoxide were the solvents tested.

Both oxidizing systems were unsatisfactory for PAH in the solid state. For PAH in solutions, only acetone proved to be satisfactory with the aqueous saturated

Table 4. Methods recommended for specific waste categories containing polycyclic aromatic hydrocarbons

Waste category	Recommended destruction method no. (in order of preference)[a]
Pure compound	1, 3, 2
Solutions in organic solvents (excluding dimethyl sulfoxide and dimethylformamide)	1, 3, 2
Solutions in dimethyl sulfoxide	2, 1, 3
Solutions in dimethylformamide	1, 3
Solutions in oil	1, 3, 2
Aqueous solutions	1
Glassware	2, 1, 3
Contents of petri dishes	1, 3, 2
Spills of pure compound in solid state	1
Spills of solutions	1

[a] Method 1: Destruction of some polycyclic aromatic hydrocarbons using potassium permanganate under acidic conditions;

Method 2: Destruction of some polycyclic aromatic hydrocarbons using concentrated sulfuric acid;

Method 3: Destruction of some polycyclic aromatic hydrocarbons using an aqueous saturated potassium permanganate solution.

solution of potassium permanganate, since dimethylformamide and dimethyl sulfoxide reacted with the oxidant and reduced the efficiency. Reduced efficiency of this oxidant was also demonstrated for treatment of dibenz[*a,h*]anthracene. With potassium permanganate in sulfuric acid, degradation yields of over 99% were obtained for all PAH, whathever the solvent.

Both oxidants gave residues that were nonmutagenic to *S. typhimurium* TA100 or had mutagenic levels not exceeding four times the background level with 900 µg equivalent of original compound per plate (160).

The two methods were successfully tested by collaborative study, and their recommended usage was adopted by the collaborative group, as presented in Table 4 (161).

(ii) *Method using treatment with undiluted sulfuric acid:* This method, suggested by Dr. G. Grimmer (personal communication), was tested with PAH in the solid state and also with solutions in acetone, dimethylformamide or dimethyl sulfoxide. Best degradation yields (in excess of 99%) were obtained with solutions in dimethyl sulfoxide with a 5 : 1 ratio of sulfuric acid : dimethyl sulfoxide. No mutagenic effect was detectable for the residues in *S. typhimurium* TA100 or TA98, with or without metabolic activation.

The method was accepted after collaborative study (see Table 4 for fields of application).

3.2.5 Hydrazines

Hydrazine and its derivatives are highly reactive and undergo a number of reactions. They are particularly easy to oxidize and most studies on their persistence in the environment and on their degradation make use of this property. Since hypochlorites have been particularly recommended, this method was reinvestigated. Oxidation is also widely used in titrimetic methods for hydrazines (162), and two of these techniques, using potassium iodate and potassium permanganate, were tested for degradation. Reduction of hydrazines to amines has also been proposed (163), as outlined earlier in this Section (3.2 (ii)) using active Raney nickel. Very good results were obtained during collaborative testing of this method, and, it was therefore accepted; the field of application is presented in Table 5 (164).

Table 5. Methods recommended for specific waste categories containing hydrazines

Waste category	Recommended destruction method no. (in order of preference)[a]
Undiluted hydrazine	1, 2, 3, 4
Aqueous solutions	1, 2, 3, 4
Solutions in methanol	1, 2, 3, 4
Solutions in ethanol	2, 3, 4
Solutions in oil	1, 2
Solutions in dimethyl sulfoxide	1
Solutions in organic solvents not miscible with water	2, 3
Contents of petri dishes	1, 4
Glassware	2, 4
Other equipment	4
Spills of aqueous, methanolic, ethanolic or organic solvent solutions	3, 4, 2
Protective clothing	4
Litter and solid absorbent material	4

[a] Some methods are not applicable to all hydrazines; see the related sections before use.

Method 1: Destruction of hydrazines in laboratory wastes using nickel-aluminium alloy in potassium hydroxide solution;

Method 2: Destruction of hydrazines in laboratory wastes using potassium permanganate in sulfuric acid;

Method 3: Destruction of hydrazines in laboratory wastes using potassium iodate;

Method 4: Destruction of hydrazines in laboratory wastes using hypochlorites.

(i) *Method using potassium iodate:* This method, which has been thoroughly studied as a titration technique (165–167), has a very wide spectrum of application, since it could be employed for hydrazine, monomethyl hydrazine, 1,1-dimethylhydrazine and 1,2-dimethylhydrazine, phenylhydrazine and other compounds, such as semicarbazide hydrochloride, carbohydrazide, amino-, diamino- and triaminoguanidines, semicarbazone and isonicotinic acid hydrazide. Better than 99% efficiency of degradation was achieved, but traces of *N*-nitrosodimethylamine were formed when 1,1-dimethylhydrazine was degraded. Strong bacterial toxicity was found with all residues when tested for mutagenic activity with *S. typhimurium* TA1530, TA1535 and TA100, with and without metabolic activation; therefore, lack of mutagenic activity could not be demonstrated unequivocally. However, in view of the excellent results obtained during the collaborative study, this method was adopted. Its field of application is presented in Table 5 (164).

(ii) *Method using hypochlorites:* Sodium and calcium hypochlorites were proposed by two groups for the treatment of spills and solutions contaminated with hydrazine (168) or spills and equipment contaminated with 1,1-dimethylhydrazine (169). The method was therefore reinvestigated for degradation of these two compounds and of methylhydrazine, 1,2-dimethylhydrazine and procarbazine. Although stoichiometric quantities were found to be sufficient to degrade the compounds in less than half an hour, a four-times excess and a 12-hour reaction time were necessary to obtain nonmutagenic residues with the *S. typhimurium* strains described in the previous sections.

Under these conditions, traces of *N*-nitrosamines were formed by the method, but it gave good results in collaborative testing and was adopted (see Table 5 for specific fields of application) (164).

(iii) *Method using potassium permanganate/sulfuric acid:* When the hydrazines under study were treated for 30 min with potassium permanganate/sulfuric acid, very efficient degradation was achieved; however, small amounts of *N*-nitrosamine are formed in most cases, and since 18–20% 1,1-dimethylhydrazine are converted to *N*-nitrosodimethylamine, this method must not be used to degrade symmetrical dialkyl or diaryl hydrazines. Since potassium permanganate/sulfuric acid can degrade small amounts of volatile *N*-nitrosamines, as outlined above (3.2 (ii)), the degradation experiment was repeated, but the reaction was left to proceed overnight. Traces of volatile *N*-nitrosamines were detected only in the residual solution of degradation of methylhydrazine. No mutagenic activity was observed in the residues of degradation of methylhydrazine, 1,1-dimethylhydrazine or procarbazine when they were tested with the *S. typhimurium* strains given above; mutagenic activity equivalent to three times the background level of spontaneous mutants was detectable with strain TA1530 with residues of degradation of hydrazines. After a successful collaborative study, the method was adopted for the degradation of methylhydrazine, 1,1-dimethylhydrazine and procarbazine and, with some reservations, for hydrazine (see Table 5 for field of application) (164).

3.2.6 Aromatic Amines

In view of the industrial importance of this class of compounds, several studies to evaluate methods of degradation of some aromatic amines in aqueous wastes and spillage have been performed and published in the literature.

Schmitt and Cagle (170) used an aqueous solution of 1% sulfuric acid and 0.5% surfactant to clean surfaces contaminated with 4,4'-methylene bis(2-chloroaniline) (MOCA). Spraying with an aqueous solution containing 5% tetrapotassium pyrophosphate and 10% sodium ethyl hexyl sulfate was proposed by Hackman and Rust (171) to remove 3,3'-dichlorobenzidine from surfaces, and the washes were further treated by diazotization. Diazotization was also used by Genin (172) to treat industrial effluents containing benzidine. Two similar methods were investigated and are discussed below.

Ozonation has been proved to be efficient for degrading benzidine and 2-naphthylamine in aqueous media (173–174), and loss of mutagenic effect was observed. In other oxidation methods that have been evaluated (175–182), the amines are oxidized to quinone imines, which can easily be reduced back to the original amines by, for example, ascorbic acid (176). The most promising oxidation technique seems to be use of potassium permanganate/sulfuric acid, and this method was investigated further (183) for a number of amines, including 4-nitrobiphenyl, a metabolite of 4-aminobiphenyl.

Oxidation of aromatic amines by hydrogen peroxide, catalysed by horseradish peroxidase (184), has also been investigated and is outlined below.

Pliss (185) showed that bromination could degrade 3,3'-dichlorobenzidine, and this method might be useful for decontamination of other aromatic amines.

(i) *Methods using diazotization:* In the early 1900s, May (186) demonstrated that diazotization in the presence of hypophosphorous acid leads to deamination. This method was investigated with 4-aminobiphenyl, benzidine, 3,3'-dichlorobenzidine, dimethylbenzidine, dimethoxybenzidine, MOCA, 1-naphthylamine, 2-naphthylamine, and *m*-toluenediamine. Better than 99% deamination of all these compounds was achieved; however, when the residues were tested for mutagenic activity, in *S. typhimurium* TA97, TA98 and TA100, with and without metabolic activation, only those of 4-aminobiphenyl were without mutagenic effect. Weak mutagenic effects were observed for degradation products of benzidine, 3,3'-dichlorobenzidine, dimethylbenzidine and dimethoxybenzidine, and up to 60 times the background level of spontaneous revertants for the degradation products of 1-naphthylamine, 2-naphthylamine, and *m*-toluenediamine. After successful collaborative study, the method was accepted for some compounds with some reserves [see Table 6 for fields of application (187)].

Using the diazotization technique proposed by Hackman and Rust (171) for the treatment of 3,3'-dichlorobenzidine, Lafontaines' group (187) investigated benzidine, dimethylbenzidine, dimethoxybenzidine, 1-naphthylamine, and *m*-toluenediamine and again 3,3'-dichlorobenzidine. Complete degradation was achieved for all these compounds, but strong mutagenic effects with the *S. typhimurium* strains described above were detected with residues from 3,3'-dichlorobenzidine, dimethoxybenzidine, 1-naphthylamine, and *m*-toluenediamine. The method was, therefore recommended for use with MOCA, benzidine and dimethylbenzidine. Its applicability is listed in Table 6.

(ii) *Methods using oxidation with potassium permanganate/sulfuric acid:* When residues of these nine aromatic amines after oxidation with potassium permanganate/sulfuric acid were analysed by ultraviolet spectrophotometry, Barek et al. (180–182) found a degrad-

59

Table 6. Methods recommended for specific waste categories containing aromatic amines or 4-nitrobiphenyl

Waste categories	Recommended destruction method no. (in order of preference)[a]	
	Aromatic amines	4-Nitro- biphenyl
Solid compound	1, 5, 3	4
Solutions in volatile organic solvents	1, 5, 3	4
Solutions in methanol	5, 3[b]	4
Solutions in ethanol	5, 3[b]	
Solutions in dimethyl sulfoxide	5, 3[b]	
Solutions in dimethylformamide	5, 3[b]	
Contents of petri dishes	2	
Solutions in water-miscible solvents	5, 3[b]	
Aqueous solutions	1, 5, 3[b]	4
Solutions in oil	1, 5, 3	
Glassware	1, 3	4
Spills of solid compounds	1, 3	
Spills of aqueous solutions	1, 3	
Spills of solutions in water-miscible solvents	3	
Spills of solutions in water-immiscible solvents (except oil)	1, 3	

[a] Some methods are not applicable to all aromatic amines tested. See related sections in the text.
   Method 1: Destruction of aromatic amines using potassium permanganate in sulfuric acid;
   Method 2: Removal of aromatic amines using horseradish peroxidase;
   Method 3: Deamination of aromatic amines by diazotization in the presence of hypophosphorous acid;
   Method 4: Destruction of 4-nitrobiphenyl using potassium permanganate in sulfuric acid;
   Method 5: Destruction of aromatic amines using diazotization.
[b] Large volumes of waste may be treated by Method 2.

ation efficiency of >99% for 3,3′-dichlorobenzidine, dimethylbenzidine, dimethoxybenzidine, benzidine and 4-aminobiphenyl, and 50% for *m*-toluenediamine, 70% for MOCA, 95% for 2-naphthylamine and 80% for 1-naphthylamine. After a slight alteration of the oxidation conditions, the residues were analysed by high-performance liquid chromatography coupled to a variable-wavelenght, ultraviolet spectrophotometric detection system and also tested for mutagenicity with the *S. typhimurium* strains. More than 99.8% degradation was achieved in all cases, and all residues were nonmutagenic. After successful collaborative study, the method was adopted as first choice for all the fields of application in which it was proposed (see Table 6) (187).

4-nitrobiphenyl proved to be poorly soluble in potassium permanganate/sulfuric acid, and direct oxidation was therefore impossible. This compound can be easily dissolved in glacial acetic acid and then reduced quantitatively to 4-aminobiphenyl by zinc powder in the presence of sulfuric acid; after filtration of the mixture to remove the zinc, addition of potassium permanganate solution allows complete degradation of 4-aminobiphenyl into nonmutagenic compounds. After successful collaborative testing, the method was adopted (see Table 6).

(iii) *Methods using oxidation by hydrogen peroxide in the presence of horseradish peroxidase:* During this catalysed oxidation, radicals were generated that could polymerize into non-water-soluble compounds. Benzidine, dimethylbenzidine dimethoxybenzidine, 3,3′-dichlorobenzidine, 1- and 2-naphthylamine can be effectively removed by this technique, but variable results were obtained with 4-aminobiphenyl. None of the solutions exerted mutagenic activity, but residues

61

of benzidine, 3,3'-dichlorobenzidine, dimethoxybenzidine and 2-naphthylamine dissolved in dimethyl sulfoxide were mutagenic. The group that took part in the validation study therefore recommended this method only for concentration of aromatic amines from large volumes of aqueous solutions.

3.2.7 Haloethers

Since recognition of the carcinogenicity of bis(chloromethyl)ether (BCME), its production has been drastically reduced; but chloromethylmethylether (CMME), which is still in use, is often contaminated by BCME. The development of safe methods for the degradation of these compounds was therefore necessary. Ammonia and other alkaline agents have been proposed for the chemical degradation of BCME (188); the efficiency of the former compound was retested, and two other methods used as derivatization techniques in the analysis of these products (189–191) were also investigated.

(i) *Method using ammonia:* In the published procedure for degradation of BCME by ammonia, a reaction time of 5 min was proposed. This was confirmed when the degradation mixtures were analysed by direct-injection gas chromatography. However, when headspace gas-chromatography-mass spectrometry was used, Telling (unpublished results) demonstrated that 3 hours were necessary to achieve better than 99.5% destruction. When the residues of treatment of CMME were tested by this latter method, less than 5 min were necessary for complete degradion; however, since CMME often contains BCME, a 3-hour reaction time was recommended. No mutagenic activity was seen when the residues were tested in *S. typhimurium* TA1530,

Table 7. Methods recommended for specific waste categories containing haloethers

Waste category	Recommended decontamination method no. (in order of preference)[a]
Undiluted compound	1, 2, 3
Solutions in organic solvents miscible with water	1, 2, 3
Solutions in organic solvents not miscible with water	1, 2, 3[b]
Solutions in solvents miscible with methanol	1, 2, 3[c]
Solutions in solvents partially miscible with methanol	1, 2, 3[b]
Glassware and solid material	1, 2, 3
Laboratory clothing	1
Spills	1

[a] Method 1: Destruction of CMME and BCME in laboratory wastes using aqueous ammonia;
Method 2: Destruction of CMME and BCME in laboratory wastes using sodium phenate;
Method 3: Destruction of CMME and BCME in laboratory wastes using sodium methoxide.
[b] Not to be used with chloroform.
[c] Not to be used in the presence of water.

TA1535 and TA100. After successful collaborative testing, the method was adopted for the applications described in Table 7 (192).

(ii) *Method using sodium methoxide or sodium phenoxide:* Alkaline metal salts of lower alcohols and phenols have been used to prepare ether derivatives quantitatively for analysis by gas chromatography. Two of them, sodium methoxide and sodium phenoxide, were tested as degradation agents for BCME and CMME; in all cases, the residues were nonmutagenic when tested with the *S. typhimurium strains* given above.

The two methods gave good results in the collaborative study and were adopted (see Table 7 for fields of application) (192).

3.2.8 Some Antineoplastic Agents

Some cancer chemotherapeutic drugs are carcinogenic and/or mutagenic. They are widely used in hospital and laboratories, and there is a widespread demand for methods for their safe disposal and for surface decontamination, a field completely neglected. Research was therefore initiated on a number of these compounds: doxorubicin, daunorubicin, methotrexate, dichloromethotrexate, cyclophosphamide, ifosfamide, vincristine sulfate, vinblastine sulfate, 6-thioguanine, 6-mercaptopurine, cisplatin, lomustine, chlorozotocin, streptozotocin, carmustine, semustine, PCNU and melphalan.

Fifteen methods were proposed and tested by collaborative study; 12 were retained, the others being rejected on the basis of mutagenic activity of the residues. Methods were approved for only the first 14 compounds and these did not cover all possible treatments of spills. The methods investigated are listed below (193).

(i) *Doxorubicin and daunorubicin:* Two methods were evaluated:

a) Oxidation with potassium permanganate (0.3 mol/L) in sulfuric acid (3 mol/L) solution: this method gave acceptable results;

b) Oxidation with 5 or 20% sodium hypochlorite solutions: this method gave acceptable chemical degradation, but was rejected on the basis of the mutagenic activity of the residues.

Table 8. Methods recommended for specific waste categories containing methotrexate or dichloromethotrexate

Waste category	Recommended destruction method no. (in order of preference)[a]	
	Metho-trexate	Dichloro-methotrexate
Solid compound	3, 4, 2	2
Aqueous solutions and pharmaceutical solutions	3, 4, 2	2
Solutions in volatile organic solvents	3, 4, 2	2
Solutions in dimethyl-formamide and dimethyl sulfoxide	2	2
Glassware	3, 4, 2	2
Spills of solid compound	4, 3, 2	2
Spills of aqueous solutions and pharmaceutical solutions	4, 3, 2	2
Spills of solutions in volatile organic solvents	4, 3, 2	2

[a] Method 2: Destruction of methotrexate and dichloromethotrexate using potassium permanganate / sulfuric acid;

Method 3: Destruction of methotrexate using aqueous alkaline potassium permanganate;

Method 4: Destruction of methotrexate using aqueous sodium hypochlorite.

(ii) *Methotrexate and dichloromethotrexate:* Three methods were evaluated:

a) Oxidation with potassium permanganate (0.3 mol/L) in sulfuric acid (3 mol/L) solution: tested with both methotrexate and dichloromethotrexate;

b) Oxidation with aqueous alkaline potassium permanganate: tested only with methotrexate;

c) Oxidation with a 30 fold excess of sodium hypochlorite solution: tested only with methotrexate.

All three methods gave acceptable results. For their fields of application, see Table 8.

(iii) *Cyclophosphamide and ifosfamide:* Three methods were evaluated. Their fields of application are given in Table 9.

a) Alkaline hydrolysis in the presence of dimethylformamide: this method gave acceptable results for both compounds;

b) Acid hydrolysis then addition of sodium thiosulfate and alkaline hydrolysis: this method gave acceptable results only for cyclophosphamide. Residues from the destruction of ifosfamide showed mutagenic activity, and the method was rejected for degradation of this compound;

c) Oxidation with potassium permanganate (0.2 mol/L) in sulfuric acid (0.5 mol/L) solution: this method resulted in acceptable chemical destruction of both compounds but was rejected on the basis of high mutagenic activity in the residues.

(iv) *Vincristine sulfate and vinblastine sulfate:* The only method tested, oxidation with potassium permanganate (0.3 mol/L) in sulfuric acid (3 mol/L) solution, gave acceptable results.

(v) *6-Thioguanine and 6-mercaptopurine:* The only method tested, oxidation with potassium permanganate (0.04 mol/L) in sulfuric acid (3 mol/L) solution, gave acceptable results.

Table 9. Methods recommended for specific waste categories containing cyclophosphamide or ifosfamide

Waste category	Recommended destruction method no.[a] (no preference)	
	Cyclophosphamide	Ifosfamide
Solid compounds	5 or 6	5
Aqueous solutions and pharmaceutical preparations	5 or 6	5
Solutions in dimethylformamide	5 or 6	5
Solutions in volatile organic solvents	5 or 6	5
Solutions in dimethyl sulfoxide	5 or 6	5
Glassware	5 or 6	5
Spills of solid compounds	5 or 6	5
Spills of aqueous solutions or of solutions in dimethylformamide or dimethyl sulfoxide	5 or 6	5
Spills of solutions in colatile organic solvents	5 or 6	5

[a] Method 5: Destruction of cyclophosphamide and ifosfamide using alkaline hydrolysis in the presence of dimethylformamide;

Method 6: Destruction of cyclophosphamide using acid hydrolysis then addition of sodium thiosulfate and alkaline hydrolysis.

(vi) *Cisplatin:* Three methods were evaluated. Their fields of application are given in Table 10.

a) Reduction with zinc powder: this method gave acceptable results;

b) Reaction with sodium diethyldithiocarbamate: no analytical method was found suitable to verify the

Table 10. Methods recommended for specific waste categories containing cisplatin

Waste category	Recommended destruction method no. (in order of preference)[a]
Solid compound	10, 9
Aqueous solutions and pharmaceutical solutions	10, 9
Solutions in water miscible solvents	9
Glassware	10, 9
Spills	10

[a] Method 9: Destruction of cisplatin by reduction with zinc powder;
Method 10: Destruction of cisplatin by reaction with sodium diethyldithiocarbamate.

level of destruction; however, no mutagenic activity was detected in the residues and the method was accepted on this basis;

c) Oxidation with potassium permanganate (0.02, 0.1 and 0.3 mol/L) in sulfuric acid solution (3 mol/L): no analytical method was found suitable to verify the level of destruction. The residues showed high mutagenic activity, and the method was therefore rejected.

(vii) *N-nitrosourea drugs:* Two methods were evaluated. Their fields of application are given in Table 11.

a) Cleavage with hydrobromic acid in glacial acetic acid: this method gave acceptable results for lomustine, chlorozotocin and streptozotocin. Destruction of PCNU was not reproducible, and the residues from treatment of carmustine and semustine showed mutagenic activity;

Table 11. Methods recommended for specific waste categories containing chlorozotocin, streptozotocin or lomustine

Waste category	Recommended destruction method no. (in order of preference)[a]		
	Chlorozotocin	Streptozotocin	Lomustine
Solid compound	11	11, 12	11
Pharmaceutical preparations (solids)	11	11, 12	11
Aqueous solutions		12	11
Pharmaceutical solutions		12	
Solutions in volatile organic solvents	11	11, 12	11
Solutions in dimethylformamide or dimethyl sulfoxide		12	
Solutions in ethanol or methanol	11	12, 11	11
Glassware	11	11, 12	11
Spills of solid compound	11	11, 12	11
Spills of liquid or pharmaceutical preparations		12	
Spills of solutions in volatile organic solvents	11	11, 12	11

[a] Method 11: Destruction of lomustine, chlorozotocin and streptozotocin using hydrobromic acid in glacial acetic acid;

Method 12: Destruction of streptozotocin using potassium permanganate / sulfuric acid.

b) Oxidation with a saturated solution of potassium permanganate in 3 mol/L sulfuric acid solution of either the pure compound or of solutions in dimethylformamide or dimethyl sulfoxide. The method was satisfactory only for streptozotocin. Chemical destruction of lomustine, carmustine, semustine, PCNU and chlorozotocin, was satisfactory, but the method was rejected on the basis of mutagenic activity of the residues.

It should be noted that, except for streptozocin, no method was validated in this study for the treatment of aqueous spills.

(viii) *Melphalan:* The only method tested, oxidation with potassium permanganate (0.3 mol/L) in sulfuric acid (3 mol/L) solution, gave satisfactory chemical destruction but was rejected on the basis of high mutagenic activity of the residues.

3.3 Conclusion

The methods presented above were tested with only a limited number of compounds. They may be applicable to other compounds of the same class, however, in each case, the efficiency of the method should first be verified, since the treatment may lead to biologically active residues. For example, denitrosation with hydrobromic acid in glacial acetic acid gave satisfactory results with eight *N*-nitrosamines and five *N*-nitrosamides, including simple *N*-nitrosoureas, but when applied to six *N*-nitrosourea drugs, it proved to be suitable for only three compounds. Similarly, diazotization was effective for some aromatic amines, but with others highly mutagenic residues were obtained.

All of the methods were tested with small quantities similar to those handled at the laboratory scale. Some may be usable for much larger quantities, but it should be borne in mind, when dealing with larger amounts, that degradation efficiency may be impaired and that even with methods with an efficiency greater than 99%

significant quantities of carcinogenic compounds may remain.

It should also be noted that a change in matrix may lead to significant changes in destruction efficiency. This is particularly true in the case of oxidation methods, in which other compounds in the medium may consume the oxidant, thus inhibiting the efficiency of degradation of the carcinogen. For example, anti-neoplastic agents are often dissolved in dextrose or mannitol solutions, which consume considerable amounts of oxidizing agents.

The chemical methods of degradation described in Section 3.2 address a wide range of solutions, and a number of them are suitable for treatment of spillage. However, only a few are useful for the treatment of bulk quantities of lightly contaminated wastes from biological experiments; for these, incineration is, at present, the only method, although biodegradation techniques may be useful.

It has not been feasible to find a universal reagent that will degrade all chemical carcinogens. Potassium permanganate/sulfuric acid oxidation was shown to be efficient for the destruction of aflatoxins, some N-nitrosamines and N-nitrosamides, some polycyclic aromatic hydrocarbons, some aromatic amines, somes hydrazines and certain antineoplastic agents, such as doxorubicin and daunorubicin, methotrexate and dichloromethotrexate, vincristine sulfate and vinblast-ine sulfate, 6-thioguanine, 6-mercaptopurine and streptozotocin, but failed under the conditions em-ployed when applied to destruction of melphalan, lomustine, carmustine, semustine, PCNU, chlorozo-tocin, cyclophosphamide and ifosfamide, cisplatin and melphalan, and when used with e. g., dialkyl- and

71

diarylhydrazines, produced large quantities of carcinogens, in this case *N*-nitrosamines. Further work is required to improve the conditions of oxidation of these compounds until nonmutagenic residues are obtained. Work will also be necessary to expand the spectrum of application of this method to other compounds of the classes covered here and to other classes of compounds. This method could, however, be useful for laboratories working simultaneously with several carcinogenic compounds.

It is hoped that an increasing number of laboratories will not only become conscious of the potential usefulness of chemical degradation techniques for decontamination of small quantities of wastes, but will also devote some time to evaluating methods for the destruction of other compounds, with a general aim of improving safety. Publication of their results should not be confined to a limited audience but should be available to all scientists and widely circulated among the public.

Acknowledgements

The authors wish to thank the Division of Safety of the National Institute of Health of the USA for their sustained support to this programme, and the following scientists for their participation at various levels in the programme of destruction of chemical carcinogens, either in the elaboration of methods or in their validation:

J. Adams
Department of Pharmacy & Chemotherapy Research
University of Texas System Cancer Center
M. D. Anderson Hospital & Tumor Institute
6723 Bertner Avenue
Houston, TX 77030, USA

M. Alvarez
Chemical Research & Development Center
FMC Corporation
Princeton, NJ 08540, USA

M. A. Armour
Department of Chemistry
The University of Alberta
Edmonton, Alberta T6G 2G2, Canada

J. Barek
Department of Analytical Chemistry
Charles University
Albertov 2030
12840 Prague 2, Czechoslovakia

M. Benard
Ecole National Supérieure des Industries
Agricoles et Alimentaires
Centre de Douai
105 rue de l'Université
59509 Douai, France

J. Benvenuto
Department of Pharmacy & Chemotherapy
Research
University of Texas System Cancer Center
M. D. Anderson Hospital & Tumor Institute
6723 Bertner Avenue
Houston, TX 77030, USA

L. van Broekhoven
Center for Agrobiological Research
P.O. Box 14
6700 AA Wageningen, The Netherlands

C. Confalonieri
Pharmaceutical Research & Development
Farmitalia Carlo Erba
Via Carlo Imbonati 24
20159 Milan, Italy

J. Dennis
Ministry of Agriculture, Fisheries & Food
Haldin House

Old Bank of England Court
Queen Street
Norwich NR2 4SX, UK

G. Eisenbrand (present address)
Department of Chemistry & Environmental
Toxicology
University of Kaiserslautern
6750 Kaiserslautern, FRG

H. P. van Egmond
National Institute of Public Health
P.O. Box 1
3720 BA Bilthoven, The Netherlands

G. Ellen
National Institute of Public Health
P.O. Box 1
3720 BA Bilthoven, The Netherlands

D. Fine
Thermedics Inc.
470 Wildwood Street
Woburn, MA 01888-1799, USA

U. Goff
Thermedics Inc.
470 Wildwood Street
Woburn, MA 01888-1799, USA

G. Grimmer
Biochemisches Institut für Umweltcarcinoge-
ne
Sieker Landstraße 19
207 Ahrensburg/Holst., FRG

D. G. Hunt
Laboratory of the Government Chemist
Cornwall House
Stamford Street
London SE1 9NQ, UK

O. Hutzinger (present address)
Chair of Ecological Chemistry
& Geochemistry
University of Bayreuth
Postfach 3008
8580 Bayreuth, FRG

M. Iovu
Chimie Organica
Facultatea de Farmacie
Str. Traian Vuia 6
Bucharest, Rumania

W. Karcher
Petten Establishment, Joint Research Center
Commission of the European Communities
P.O. Box 2
1755 ZG Petten, The Netherlands

L. K. Keefer (present address)
Laboratory of Comparative Carcinogenesis
Division of Cancer Etiology
National Cancer Institute
Frederick, MD 21701, USA

D. Klein (present address)
Centre de Recherche Crealis
Rue Frédéric Sauvage
19100 Brive La Gaillarde, France

M. Klibanov
Department of Nutrition & Food Science
Massachusetts Institute of Technology
Cambridge, MA 02139, USA

H. Kunte
Hygiene Institut
Hochhaus am Augusplatz
65 Mainz, FRG

M. Lafontaine
Institut National de Recherche et de Sécurité
Service Chimie Toxicologique
Avenue de Bourgogne
54500 Vandoeuvre, France

S. Ludeman
Department of Chemistry
The Catholic University of America
Washington DC 20064, USA

R. Massey
Ministry of Agriculture, Fisheries & Food
Haldin House
Old Bank of England Court
Queen Street
Norwich NR2 4SX, UK

R. Mitchum (present address)
Quality Assurance Division
US Environmental Protection Agency
Office of Research & Development
Environmental Monitoring Systems
Laboratory
P.O. Box 15027
Las Vegas, NV 89114, USA

H. C. van der Plas
Laboratory of Organic Chemistry
De Dreijen 5
6703 BC Wageningen, The Netherlands

D. Reed
Department of Biochemistry & Biophysics
Oregon State University
Corvallis, OR 97331, USA

P. van Roosmalen
Alberta Workers' Health,
Safety & Compensation
Laboratory Services Branch
Occupational Health & Safety Division
10158-103 Street
Edmonton, Alberta T5J OX6, Canada

P. L. Schuller (present address)
Keuringsdienst Van Waren Door Het Gehied
Evertsenstraat 17
4461 XN Goes, The Netherlands

M. G. Siriwardana (present address)
Gesira University
Wad Medani
Sudan

P. L. R Smith
British Food Manufacturers Industries
Research Association
Randalls Road
Leatherhead KT22 7RY, UK

B. Spiegelhalder
German Cancer Research Center
Institute of Toxicology & Chemotherapy
Im Neuenheimer Feld 280
6900 Heidelberg, FRG

D. Spincer
Imperial Group Ltd.
Raleigh Road
Bristol BS3 1QX, UK

A. Stacchini
Institute Superiore di Sanita
Viale Regina Elena 299
00161 Rome, Italy

L. A. Sternson (present address)
Pharmaceutical Research & Technologies
Chemical Research & Development
1500 Spring Garden Street
P.O. Box 7929
Philadelphia, PA 19101, USA

G. M. Telling
Unilever Research
Colworth Laboratory
Sharnbrook, Beds., MK44 1LQ, UK

S. P. Tucker
National Institute for Occupational Safety
& Health
Division of Physical Sciences & Engineering
Methods Research Branch
Organic Methods Development Section
Public Health Service

Roberts A. Taft Laboratories
4676 Columbia Parkway
Cincinnati, OH 45226, USA

M. Vahl
Ministry of Environment
National Food Institute
Statens Levensdsmiddelinstitut
Morkhoj Bygade 19
2860 Soborg, Denmark

J. J. Vallon
Laboratoire de Chimie Analytique
Pharmaceutique
Faculté de Médecine et de Pharmacie
8 Avenue Rockfeller
69008 Lyon, France

E. A. Walker (present address)
The Bowery
58 b Chestfield Road
Chestfield, Kent CT5 3JH, UK

K. Webb
Laboratory of the Government Chemist
Cornwall House
Stamford Street
London SE1 9NQ, UK

D. T. Williams
Bureau of Chemical Hazards
Environmental Health Center
Health & Welfare Canada
Tunneys Pasture
Ottawa, Ontario K1A OL2, Canada

References

1. Young, J. R.: J. Chem. Educ. *48*, A349 (1971)

2. Fawcett, H. H., Wood, W. S. (eds.): Safety and Accident Prevention in Chemical Operations, New York, Interscience, John Wiley & Sons 1965

3. Steere, N. V. (ed.): Handbook of Laboratory Safety, Cleveland, OH, The Chemical Rubber Company 1967, 1971

4. Muir, G. D. (ed.): Hazards in the Chemical Laboratory, London, The Chemical Society, 1971[1], 1977[2]

5. Bretherick, L.: Handbook of Reactive Chemical Hazards, Boca Raton, FL, The Chemical Rubber Company, 1975

6. Green, M. E., Turk, A.: Safety in Working with Chemicals, New York, MacMillan Publishing Company, 1978

7. National Research Council, National Academy of Sciences, National Academy of Engineering, Institute of Medecine: Prudent Practices for Handling Hazardous Chemicals in Laboratories, Washington DC., National Academy Press, 1981

8. Li, L. P., Fraumeni, J. F., Mantel, N., Miller, R. W.: J. Natl. Cancer Inst., *43*, 1159 (1969)

9. Olin, R.: Lancet, ii, 916 (1976)

10. Olin, R.: J. Am. Ind. Hyg. Assoc., *39*, 557 (1978)

11. Searle, C. E., Waterhouse, J. A. H., Henman, B. A., Bartlett, D., McCombie, S.: Br. J. Cancer, *38*, 192 (1978)

12. Olsson, H., Brandt, L.: Br. Med. J., *ii*, 580 (1981)

13. Olin, G. R., Ahlbom, A.: Environ. Res., *22*, 154 (1980)

14. Austin, D. F., Reynolds, P. J., Snyder, M. A., Biggs, M. W., Stubbs, H. A.: Lancet, *ii*, 712 (1981)

15. Hoar, S. K., Pell, S.: J. Occup. Med., *23*, 485 (1981)

16. Meston, M. C.: Code of Practice for the Handling, Storage and Use of Chemical Carcinogens, Mutagens and Teratogens, University of Aberdeen

17. Chester Beatty Research Institute: Precautions for Laboratory Workers who Handle Carcinogenic Amines, London, 1971

18. National Institute of Health (USA): National Cancer Institute Safety Standards for Research involving Chemical Carcinogens (DHEW Publication No. 75–900), Bethesda, MD, 1975

19. Medical Research Council (UK): Guidelines for Work with Chemical Carcinogens in Medical Research Council Establishments, London, 1979

20. National Center for Toxicological Research (USA): NCTR Carcinogen Standards, Jefferson, AR, 1975

21. Loogna, G. O., Kann, Y. M.: Safety measures in handling N-nitroso compounds, in: proceedings of the Second Symposium on Carcinogenic N-Nitroso Compounds: Action, Synthesis, Detection, p. 122, Tallin, 1975

22. Searle, C. E.: Chem. Br. *6*, 5 (1970)

23. Cater, D. B., Hartree, E.: Biochem. Soc. Spec. Publ., *5*, 47 (1977)

24. Montesano, R., Bartsch, H., Boyland, E., Della Porta, G., Fishbein, L., Griesemer, R. A., Swan, A. B., Tomatis, L. (eds.): Handling Chemical Carcinogens in the Laboratory, Problems of Safety. (IARC Scientific Publications No. 33), Lyon, International Agency for Research on Cancer, 1979

25. National Institutes of Health (USA): NIH Guidelines for the Laboratory Use of Chemical Carcinogens, Washington DC, 1981

26. Le Neveu, D. M., Hawkins, R. J., Weeks, J. L.: A Guide to Safe Handling of Non-radioactive Chemical Carcinogens in the Laboratory, Pinawa, Manitoba, Health & Safety Division, Whiteshell Nuclear Research Establishment, Atomic Energy of Canada Limited, 1980

27. New York University Medical Center: Chemical Carcinogens Safety Regulations, New York, 1981

28. Nemoto, N.: Hen'igen do Dokusei, *4*, 18 (1981)

29. Sferazza, G.: Inquinamento, *6*, 115 (1980)

30. Picot, A.: Actual. Chimique, 25 (Mars 1983)

31. Songer, J. R. & Braymen, D. T.: Safe use and disposal of hazardous chemicals in the laboratory, in: Thin Layer Chromatography: Quantitative Environmental and Clinical Applications (eds.) J. C. Touchstone, D. Rogers, Chapter 24, New York, John Wiley and Sons, 1980

32. Fleischhauer, G.: Ber. Int. Kollog. Verhuetung Arbeitson Faellen Berofskr Chem. Ind., *8*, 51, 1982

33. Johnson, J. S.: Safe handling of chemical carcinogens, mutagens, teratogens and highly toxic substances, in: Safe Handling of Chemical Carcinogen in the Research Laboratory, (ed.) Walters, D. B., vol. 1, p. 139, 1980, Ann Arbor, MI, Ann Arbor Science.

34. Steere N. V.: J. Chem. Educ., *51*, A322 (1974)

35. Steere N. V.: J. Chem. Educ., *51*, A366 (1974)

36. Steere N. V.: J. Chem. Educ., *51*, A431 (1974)

37. IARC: IARC Monographs on the Evaluation of Carcinogenic Risk of Chemicals to Man, Vol. 1, Some Inorganic Substances, Chlorinated Hydrocarbons, Aromatic Amines, N-Nitroso Compounds and Natural Products, Lyon, International Agency for Research on Cancer, 1972

38. IARC: IARC Monographs on the Evaluation of Carcinogenic Risk of Chemicals to Man, Vol. 2, Some Inorganic and Organometallic Compounds, Lyon, International Agency for Research on Cancer, 1973

39. IARC: IARC Monographs on the Evaluation of Carcinogenic Risk of Chemicals to Man, Vol. 3, Certain Polycyclic Aromatic Hydrocarbons and Heterocyclic Compounds, Lyon, International Agency for Research on Cancer, 1973

40. IARC: IARC Monographs on the Evaluation of Carcinogenic Risk of Chemicals to Man, Vol. 4, Some Aromatic Amines, Hydrazine and Related Substances, *N*-Nitroso Compounds and Miscellaneous Alkylating Agents, Lyon, International Agency for Research on Cancer, 1974

41. IARC: IARC Monographs on the Evaluation of Carcinogenic Risk of Chemicals to Man, Vol. 5, Some Organochlorine Pesticides, Lyon, International Agency for Research on Cancer, 1974

42. IARC: IARC Monographs on the Evaluation of Carcinogenic Risk of Chemicals to Man, Vol. 6, Sex Hormones, Lyon, International Agency for Research on Cancer, 1974

43. IARC: IARC Monographs on the Evaluation of Carcinogenic Risk of Chemicals to Man, Vol. 7, Some Antithyroid and Related Substances, Nitrofurans and Industrial Chemicals, Lyon, International Agency for Research on Cancer, 1974

44. IARC: IARC Monographs on the Evaluation of Carcinogenic Risk of Chemicals to Man, Vol. 8, Some Aromatic Azo Compounds, Lyon, International Agency for Research on Cancer, 1975

45. IARC: IARC Monographs on the Evaluation of Carcinogenic Risk of Chemicals to Man, Vol. 9, Some Aziridines, N-, S- *and* O-Mustards and Selenium, Lyon, International Agency for Research on Cancer, 1975

46. IARC: IARC Monographs on the Evaluation of Carcinogenic Risk of Chemicals to Man, Vol. 10, Some Naturally Occurring Substances, Lyon, International Agency for Research on Cancer, 1976

47. IARC: IARC Monographs on the Evaluation of Carcinogenic Risk of Chemicals to Man, Vol. 11, Cadmium, Nickel, Some Epoxides, Miscellaneous Industrial Chemicals and General Considerations on Volatile Anaesthetics, Lyon, International Agency for Research on Cancer, 1976

48. IARC: IARC Monographs on the Evaluation of Carcinogenic Risk of Chemicals to Man, Vol. 12, Some Carbamates, Thiocarbamates and Carbazides, Lyon, International Agency for Research on Cancer, 1976

49. IARC: IARC Monographs on the Evaluation of Carcinogenic Risk of Chemicals to Man, Vol. 13, Some Miscellaneous Pharmaceutical Substances, Lyon, International Agency for Research on Cancer, 1977

50. IARC: IARC Monographs on the Evaluation of Carcinogenic Risk of Chemicals to Man, Vol. 14, Asbestos, Lyon, International Agency for Research on Cancer, 1977

51. IARC: IARC Monographs on the Evaluation of the Carcinogenic Risk of Chemicals to Man, Vol. 15, Some Fumigants, the Herbicides 2,4-D and 2,4,5-T, Chlorinated Dibenzodioxins and Miscellaneous Industrial Chemicals, Lyon, International Agency for Research on Cancer, 1977

52. IARC: IARC Monographs on the Evaluation of the Carcinogenic Risk of Chemicals to Man, Vol. 16, Some Aromatic Amines, and Related Nitro Compounds: Hair Dyes, Colouring Agents and Miscellaneous Industrial Chemicals, Lyon, International Agency for Research on Cancer, 1978

53. IARC: IARC Monographs on the Evaluation of the Carcinogenic Risk of Chemicals to Humans, Vol. 17, Some N-Nitroso Compounds, Lyon, International Agency for Research on Cancer, 1978

54. IARC: IARC Monographs on the Evaluation of the Carcinogenic Risk of Chemicals to Humans, Vol. 18, Polychlorinated Biphenyls and Polybrominated Biphenyls, Lyon, International Agency for Research on Cancer, 1978

55. IARC: IARC Monographs on the Evaluation of the Carcinogenic Risk of Chemicals to Humans, Vol. 19, Some Monomers, Plastics and Synthetic Elastomers, and Acrolein, Lyon, International Agency for Research on Cancer, 1979

56. IARC: IARC Monographs on the Evaluation of the Carcinogenic Risk of Chemicals to Humans, Vol. 20, Some Halogenated Hydrocarbons, Lyon, International Agency for Research on Cancer, 1979

57. IARC: IARC Monographs on the Evaluation of the Carcinogenic Risk of Chemicals to Humans, Vol. 21, Sex Hormone (II), Lyon, International Agency for Research on Cancer, 1979

58. IARC: IARC Monographs on the Evaluation of the Carcinogenic Risk of Chemicals to Humans, Volumes 1–20, Supplement 1, Chemicals and Industrial Processes Associated with Cancer in Humans (IARC Monographs, Volumes 1 to 20), Lyon, International Agency for Research on Cancer, 1979

59. IARC: Information Bulletin on the Survey of Chemicals being Tested for Carcinogenicity Vol. 8, Lyon, International Agency for Research on Cancer, 1979

60. IARC: IARC Monographs on the Evaluation of the Carcinogenic Risk of Chemicals to Humans, Vol. 22, Some Non-nutritive Sweetening Agents, Lyon, International Agency for Research on Cancer, 1980

61. IARC: IARC Monographs on the Evaluation of the Carcinogenic Risk of Chemicals to Humans, Vol. 23, Some Metals and Metallic Compounds, Lyon, International Agency for Research on Cancer, 1980

62. IARC: IARC Monographs on the Evaluation of the Carcinogenic Risk of Chemicals to Humans, Vol. 24, Some Pharmaceutical Drugs, Lyon, International Agency for Research on Cancer, 1980

63. IARC: IARC Monographs on the Evaluation of the Carcinogenic Risk of Chemicals to Humans, Vol. 25, Wood Leather and some associated Industries, Lyon, International Agency for Research for Cancer, 1981

64. IARC: IARC Monographs on the Evaluation of the Carcinogenic Risk of Chemicals to Humans, Vol. 26, Some Antineoplastic an Immunosuppressive Agents, Lyon, International Agency for Research for Cancer, 1981

65. IARC: IARC Monographs on the Evaluation of the Carcinogenic Risk of Chemicals to Humans, Vol. 27, Some Aromatic Amines, Anthraquinones and Nitroso Compounds, and Inorganic Fluorides used in Drinking-water and Dental Preparations, Lyon, International Agency for Research on Cancer, 1982

66. IARC: IARC Monographs on the Evaluation of the Carcinogenic Risk of Chemicals to Humans, Vol. 28, The Rubber Industry, Lyon, International Agency for Research on Cancer, 1982

67. IARC: IARC Monographs on the Evaluation of the Carcinogenic Risk of Chemicals to Humans, Vol. 29, Some Industrial Chemicals and Dyestuffs, Lyon, International Agency for Research on Cancer, 1982

68. IARC: IARC Monographs on the Evaluation of the Carcinogenic Risk of Chemicals to Humans. Supplement

No. 4, Chemicals, Industrial Processes and Industries Associated with Cancer in Humans (IARC Monographs, Volumes 1–29), Lyon, International Agency for Research on Cancer, 1982

69. IARC: IARC Monographs on the Evaluation of the Carcinogenic Risk of Chemicals to Humans, Vol. 30, Miscellaneous Pesticides, Lyon, International Agency for Research on Cancer, 1983

70. IARC: IARC Monographs on the Evaluation of the Carcinogenic Risk of Chemicals to Humans, Vol. 31, Some Food Additives, Feed Additives and Naturally Occurring Substances, Lyon, International Agency for Research on Cancer, 1983

71. IARC: IARC Monographs on the Evaluation of the Carcinogenic Risk of Chemicals to Humans, Vol. 32, Polynuclear Aromatic Compounds, Part 1, Chemical, Environmental and Experimental Data, Lyon, International Agency for Research on Cancer, 1984

72. IARC: IARC Monographs on the Evaluation of the Carcinogenic Risk of Chemicals to Humans, Vol. 33, Polynuclear Aromatic Compounds, Part 2, Carbon Blacks, Mineral Oils and Some Nitroarene Compounds, Lyon, International Agency for Research on Cancer, 1984

73. IARC: IARC Monographs on the Evaluation of the Carcinogenic Risk of Chemicals to Humans, Vol. 34, Polynuclear Aromatic Compounds, Part 3, Industrial Exposures in Aluminium Production, Coal Gasification, Coke Production and Iron and Steel Founding, Lyon, International Agency for Research on Cancer, 1984

74. Keith, L. H., Harless, J. M., Walters, D. B.: Analysis and storage of hazardous environmental chemicals for toxicological testing, in: Environmental Health Chemistry of Environmental Agents as Potential Human Hazards (eds.) McKinney, J. D., Ann Arbor, MI, Ann Arbor Science, 1981

75. International Air Transport Association (IATA): Dangerous Good Regulations, Montreal, 1984

76. Rappaport, S. M., Campbell, E. E.: Am. Ind. Hyg. Assoc. J., *37*, 690 (1976)

77. Johnson, J. S.: Safe handling of chemical carcinogen in the research laboratory, in: Safe Handling of Chemical Carcinogens, Mutagens, Teratogens and Highly Toxic Substances (ed.), Walters, D. B., Vol. 1, p. 139, Ann Arbor, MI, Ann Arbor Science, 1980

78. Barbeito, M. S.: ACS Symp. Ser. *79*, 191 (1979)

79. Meiners, A. F., Reisdorf, R. P., Owens, H. P.: Carcinogen spills: A challenge to laboratory safety capability, in: Safe Handling of Chemical Carcinogens, Mutagens, Teratogens and Highly Toxic Substances (ed.), Walters, D. B., Volume 2, p. 509, Ann Arbor, MI, Ann Arbor Science, 1980

80. Ehrenberg, L., Wachtmeister, C. A.: Safety precautions in work with mutagenic and carcinogenic chemicals, in: Handbook of Mutagenicity Test Procedures (eds.) Kilbey, B. J., Legator, M., Nicols, W., Ramel, C., p. 401, Amsterdam, Elsevier, 1977

81. Sansone, E. B., Wodchow, H., Chatigny, M. A., Anal. Chem., *49*, 670 (1977)

82. Huberman, E., Traut, M., Sachs, L.: J. Natl. Cancer Inst., *44*, 395 (1970)

83. Sansone, E. B., Losikoff, A. M., Pendleton, R. A.: J. Am. Ind. Hyg. Assoc., *38*, 433 (1977)

84. Sansone, E. B., Losikoff, A. M.: J. Am. Ind. Hyg. Assoc., *40*, 543 (1979)

85. Preussmann, R., Castegnaro, M., Walker, E. A., Wasserman, A. (eds.): Environmental Carcinogens. Selected Methods of Analysis, Vol. 1, Analysis of Volatile Nitrosamines in Food (IARC Scientific Publications No. 18), Lyon, International Agency for Research on Cancer, 1978

86. Squirell, D. C. M., Thain, W. (eds.): Environmental Carcinogens. Selected Methods of Analysis, Vol. 2, Methods for the Measurement of Vinyl Chloride in Poly(vinyl chloride), Air, Water and Foodstuffs (IARC Scientific Publications No. 22), Lyon, International Agency for Research on Cancer, 1978

87. Castegnaro, M., Bogovski, P., Kunte, H., Walker, E. A. (eds.): Environmental Carcinogens. Selected Methods of Analysis, Vol. 3, Analysis of Polycyclic Aromatic Hydro-

carbons in Environmental Samples (IARC Scientific Publications No. 29), Lyon, International Agency for Research on Cancer, 1979

88. Fishbein, L., Castegnaro, M., O'Neill, I. K., Bartsch, H. (eds.): Environmental Carcinogens. Selected Methods of Analysis, Vol. 4, Some Aromatic Amines and Azo Dyes in the General and Industrial Environment (IARC Scientific Publications No. 40), Lyon, International Agency for Research on Cancer, 1981

89. Stoloff, L., Castegnaro, M., Scott, P., O'Neill, I. K., Bartsch, H. (eds.): Environmental Carcinogens. Selected Methods of Analysis, Vol. 5, Some Mycotoxins (IARC Scientific Publications No. 44), Lyon, International Agency for Research on Cancer, 1984

90. Preussmann, R., O'Neill, I. K., Eisenbrand, G., Spiegelhalder, B., Bartsch, H. (eds.): Environmental Carcinogens. Selected Methods of Analysis, Vol. 6, N-Nitroso Compounds (IARC Scientific Publications No. 45), Lyon, International Agency for Research on Cancer, 1984

91. Sansone, E. B., Fox, J. G.: Lab. Anim. Sci., 27, 457 (1977)

92. Sansone, E. B., Losikoff, A. M.: Toxicol. Appl. Pharmacol., 46, 703 (1978)

93. Sansone, E. B., Losikoff, A. M.: Toxicol. Appl. Pharmacol., 50, 115 (1979)

94. Sansone, E. B., Losikoff, A. M., Pendleton, R. A.: Toxicol. Appl. Pharmacol., 39, 435 (1977)

95. Sansone, E. B., Jonas, L. A.: J. Am. Ind. Hyg. Assoc., 42, 688 (1981)

96. Gough, T. A., Webb, K. S., McPhail, M. F.: Diffusion of nitrosamines through protective gloves, in: Environmental Aspects of N-Nitroso Compounds (IARC Scientific Publications No. 19), (eds.) Walker, E. A., Castegnaro, M., Griciute, L., Lyle, L. E., p. 531, Lyon, International Agency for Research on Cancer, 1978

97. Sansone, E. B., Tewari, Y. B. (1978): The permeability of laboratory gloves to selected nitrosamines, in: Environmental Aspects of N-Nitroso Compounds (IARC Scientific Publications No. 19) (eds.) Walker, E. A., Castegnaro,

M., Griciute, L., Lyle, L. E., p. 517, Lyon, International Agency for Research on Cancer, 1978

98. Walker, E. A., Castegnaro, M., Garren, L., Pignatelli, B.: Limitation to the protective effect of rubber gloves for handling nitrosamines, in: Environmental Aspects of N-Nitroso Compounds (IARC Scientific Publications No. 19) (eds.) Walker, E. A., Castegnaro, M., Griciute, L., Lyle, L. E., p. 535, Lyon, International Agency for Research on Cancer, 1978

99. Sansone, E. B., Tewari, Y. B.: J. Am. Ind. Hyg. Assoc., 39, 169 (1978)

100. Sansone, E. B., Tewari, Y. B.: J. Am. Ind. Hyg. Assoc., 39, 921 (1978)

101. Weeks, R. W., Dean, B. J.: J. Am. Ind. Hyg. Assoc., 38, 721 (1977)

102. Castegnaro, M., van Egmond, H. P., Paulsch, W. E., Michelon, J.: J. Assoc. Off. Anal. Chem., 65, 1520 (1982)

103. Sansone, E. B., Tewari, Y. B.: J. Am. Ind. Hyg. Assoc., 41, 527 (1980)

104. Joyce, R. M.: Science, 224, 449 (1984)

105. Dwyer, J. L.: Contamination Analysis and Control, New York, Reinhold, (1966)

106. Steere, N. V. (ed.): Handbook of Laboratory Safety, Cleveland, OH, Chemical Rubber Co., 1971[1]

107. Manufacturing Chemists Association: Laboratory Waste Disposal Manual, Washington DC, 1973

108. American Institute of Chemical Engineers: Control of Hazardous Material Spills, Washington DC, 1974

109. American Chemical Society: Safety in Academic Chemistry Laboratories, Rev. ed., Washington DC, 1976

110. Rubey, W. A., Hall, D. L., Torres, J. L., Dellinger, B., Carnes, R. A.: Proceedings of the 7th International Symposium on Polynuclear Aromatic Hydrocarbons, p. 1047, Battelle, Columbus, Battelle Press, Columbus, Springer-Verlag, New York, Heidelberg, Berlin, 1983

111. Rappe, C.: Decontamination of products formed during the industrial preparation of 2,4,5-trichlorophenol, in:

Dioxin: Toxicological and Chemical Aspects (eds.) Cattabeni, F., Cavallaro, A., Galli, G., p. 179, SP Medical & Scientific Books, Halsted Press a division of John Wiley, 1978

112. Wilkinson, T. K., Rogers, H. W.: Disposal of chemical carcinogens, mutagens and teratogens from research facilities, in: safe Handling of Chemical Carcinogens, Mutagens, Teratogens and Highly Toxic Substances (ed.) Walter, D. B., p. 575, Ann Arbor, MI, Ann Arbor Science, 1980

113. Coombs, M. M., Castegnaro, M.: Low catalytic oxidation of polycyclic carcinogens, in: The Disposal of Hazardous Waste from Laboratories, p. 31, London, The Royal Society of Chemistry, 1983

114. Rosenhaft, M. E.: Lab. Anim. Sci., *24*, 905 (1974)

115. Walker, E. A., Castegnaro, M.: Nature, *284*, 210 (1980)

116. International Agency for Research on Cancer: Internal Technical Report No. 79/002, 1979

117. Ames, B. N., McCann, J., Yamasaki, E.: Mutat. Res., *31*, 347 (1975)

118. Bartsch, H., Malaveille, C., Camus, A. M., Martel-Planche, G., Brun, G., Hautefeuille, A., Sabadie, N., Barbin, A., Kuroki, T., Drevon, C., Piccoli, C., Montesano, R.: Mutat. Res., *76*, 1 (1980)

119. Fried, J.: Am. Lab., *9*, 79 (1977)

120. King, V. M.: Am. Lab., *10*, 69 (1978)

121. Detroy, R. W., Lillehoj, E. B., Ciegler, A.: Aflatoxins and related compounds, in: Microbial Toxins (eds.) Ciegler, A., Kadis, S., Ajl, S. J., p. 3–178, New York, Academic Press, 1971

122. Goldblatt, L. A., Dollear, F. G.: Pure Appl. Chem., *49*, 1759 (1977)

123. Beckwith, A. C., Vesonder, R. F., Ciegler, A.: Chemical methods investigated for detoxifying aflatoxins in foods and feeds, in: Mycotoxins and Other Fungal Related Food Problems (ed.) Rodrick, J. W., Washington DC, American Chemical Society, 1976

124. Ciegler, A.: Toxicon, *Suppl. 1*, 729 (1978)

125. Jemmali, M.: Pure Appl. Chem., *52*, 175 (1979)

126. Fischbach, H., Campbell, A. D.: J. Assoc. Off. Anal. Chem., *48*, 28 (1965)

127. Stoloff, L., Trager, W.: J. Assoc. Off. Anal. Chem., *48*, 681 (1965)

128. Trager, W., Stoloff, L.: J. Agric. Food Chem., *15*, 679 (1967)

129. Castegnaro, M., Friesen, M., Michelon, J., Walker, E. A.: Am. Ind. Hyg. Assoc. J., *42*, 398 (1981)

130. Swenson, D. H., Miller, J. S., Miller, E. C.: Cancer Res., *35*, 3811 (1975)

131. Castegnaro, M., Hunt, D. C., Sansone, E. B., Schuller, P. L., Siriwardanna, M. G., Telling, G. M., van Egmond, H. P., Walker, E. A. (eds.): Laboratory Decontamination and Destruction of Aflatoxins B_1, B_2, G_1, G_2 in Laboratory Wastes (IARC Scientific Publications No. 37), Lyon, International Agency for Research on Cancer, 1980

132. Vesonder, R. F., Beckwith, A. C., Ciegler, A., Dimler, R. J.: J. Agric. Food Chem., *23*, 242 (1975)

133. Gangolli, S. D., Shilling, W. H., Llyod, A. G.: Food Cosmet. Toxicol., *12*, 168 (1974)

134. Eizember, R. F., Vogler, K. R., Souter, R. W., Cannon, W. N., Wegge, P. M., II: J. Org. Chem., *44*, 784 (1979)

135. Ehrenberg, L., Wachtmeister, C. A.: Safety precautions in work with mutagenic and carcinogenic chemicals, in: Handbook of Mutagenicity Test Procedures (eds.) Kilberg, B. J., Legator, M., Nicols, W., Ramel, C., p. 401, Amsterdam, Elsevier, 1977

136. Chien, R. T., Thomas, M. H.: J. Environ. Pathol. Toxicol., *2*, 513 (1978)

137. Emmet, G. C., Michejda, C. J., Sansone, E. B., Keefer, L. K.: Limitation of photodegradation in the decontamination and disposal of chemical carcinogens, in: Safe Handling of Chemical Carcinogens, Mutagens, Teratogens and Highly Toxic Substances (ed.) Walter, D. B., p. 535, Ann Arbor, MI, Ann Arbor Science, 1979

138. Lunn, G., Sansone, E. B., Keefer, L. K.: Food Cosmet. Toxicol., *19*, 493 (1981)

139. Lunn, G., Sansone, E. B., Keefer, L. K.: Carcinogenesis, *4*, 315 (1983)

140. Castegnaro, M., Eisenbrand, G., Ellen, G., Keefer, L., Klein, D., Sansone, E. B., Spincer, D., Telling, G. M., Webb, K. (eds.): Laboratory Decontamination and Destruction of Carcinogens in Laboratory Wastes: Some N-Nitrosamines. (IARC Scientific Publications No. 43), Lyon, International Agency for Research on Cancer, 1982

141. Castegnaro, M., Michelon, J., Walker, E. A.: Some detoxifications methods for nitrosamine contaminated wastes, in: *N*-Nitroso Compounds: Occurrence and Biological Effects (IARC Scientific Publications No. 41), (eds.) Bartsch, H., O'Neill, I. K., Castegnaro, M., Okada, M., p. 151, Lyon, International Agency for Research on Cancer, 1982

142. Eisenbrand, G., Preussmann, R.: Arzneimittel. Forsch., *20*, 1513 (1970)

143. Johnson, E. M., Walters, C. L.: Anal. Lett., *4*, 383 (1971)

144. Hünig, S., Geldern, L., Lücke, E.: Angew. Chem. *75*, 476 (1963)

145. Castegnaro, M., Pignatelli, B., Walker, E. A.: An investigation of the possible value of oxonium salt formation in nitrosamine analysis, in: *N*-Nitroso Compounds in the Environment (IARC Scientific Publications No. 9), (eds.) Bogovski, P., Walker, E. A., p. 45, Lyon, International Agency for Research on Cancer, 1974

146. Lobl, T. J.: J. Chem. Educ., *49*, 730 (1972)

147. Douglas, M. L., Kabacoff, B. L., Anderson, J. A., Cheng, M. C.: J. Soc. Cosmet. Chem., *29*, 581 (1978)

148. Lunn, G., Sansone, E. B., Andrews, A. W., Castegnaro, M., Malaveille, C., Michelon, J., Brouet, I., Keefer, L.: Destruction of carcinogenic and mutagenic N-nitrosamides in laboratory wastes, in: *N*-Nitroso Compounds: Occurrence Biological Effects and Relevance to Human Cancer (IARC Scientific Publications No. 57) (eds.) O'Neill, I. K., von Borstel, R. C., Miller, C. T., Long,

93

J., Bartsch, H., p. 387, Lyon, International Agency for Research on Cancer, 1983

149. Castegnaro, M., Benard, M., Van Broekhoven, L. W., Fine, D., Massey, R., Sansone, E. B., Smith, P. L. R., Spiegelhalder, B., Stacchini, A., Telling, G., Vallon, J. J. (eds.): Laboratory Decontamination and Destruction of Carcinogens in Laboratory Wastes: Some N-Nitrosamides (IARC Scientific Publications No. 55), Lyon, International Agency for Research on Cancer, 1983

150. Grochmalicka, M. J., Okoda, J. R., Lulek, J.: Gaz Woda. Techn. Sanit., 53, 74 (1979)

151. Shkodich, P. E., Gracheua, M. P., Tikhomirov, Ya. P., Baikovsky, V. V.: Gig. Sanit., 40, 13–15 (1975)

152. Shkodich, P. E., Baikovsky, V. V., Korolev, A. A., Tikhomirov, Y. P.: Vodn. Resur., 3, 132 (1977)

153. Trakhtman, N. N., Manita, M. D.: Gig. Sanit., 31, 316 (1966)

154. Graaf, W., Nothhafft, G.: Arch. Hyg. Bakteriol., 147, 135 (1963)

155. Reichert, J. K.: Arch. Hyg. Bakteriol., 152, 37 (1968)

156. Reichert, J. K.: Arch. Hyg. Bakteriol., 152, 265 (1968)

157. Reichert, J. K.: Arch. Hyg. Bakteriol., 152, 277 (1968)

158. Malik, M., Cooke, M. F., Guyer, G. M., Semenivk, G. M., Sawicki, E.: Anal. Lett., 8, 511 (1975)

159. Tipson, R. S.: Oxidation of Polycyclic Aromatic Hydrocarbons (NBS Publication No. 87), Washington DC, (1965)

160. Castegnaro, M., Coombs, M., Phillipson, M. A., Bourgade, M. C., Michelon, J.: The use of potassium permanganate for the detoxification of some PAH contaminated wastes, in: Proceedings of the 7th Symposium on Polynuclear Hydrocarbons, p. 257, Battelle Columbus Laboratories, Battelle press, Columbus, Springer Verlag, New York, Heidelberg, Berlin, 1983

161. Castegnaro, M., Grimmer, G., Hutzinger, O., Karcher, W., Kunte, H., Lafontaine, M., Sansone, E. B., Telling, G., Tucker, S. P. (eds.): Laboratory Decontamination and

Destruction of Carcinogens in Laboratory Wastes: Some Polycyclic Aromatic Hydrocarbons (IARC Scientific Publications No. 49), Lyon, International Agency for Research on Cancer, 1983

162. Malone, H. G.: The Determination of Hydrazino-Hydrazide Groups, Pergamon Press, p. 1, New York, 1970

163. Lunn, G., Sansone, E. B., Keefer, L. K.: Environ. Sci. Technol., *17*, 240 (1983)

164. Castegnaro, M., Ellen, G., Lafontaine, M., van der Plas, H. C., Sansone, E. B., Tucker, S. P. (eds.): Laboratory Decontamination and Destruction of Carcinogens in Laboratory Wastes: Some Hydrazines (IARC Scientific Publications No. 54), Lyon, International Agency for Research on Cancer, 1983

165. Miller, G. O., Furman, N. H.: J. Am. Chem. Soc., *59*, 161 (1937)

166. McBride, W. R., Henry, R. A., Skolnick, S.: Anal. Chem., *25*, 1042 (1953)

167. McBride, W. R., Kruse, H. W.: Anal. Chem., *79*, 572 (1956)

168. Stauffer, T. B., Eyl, A. W.: Studies on Evaporation of Hydrazines and Procedure for Clean-up of Small Spills (Report CEEDO-TR-78-12), Tyndall Air Force Base, FL, Civil and Engineering Development Office, 1978

169. Mach, M. H., Baumgartner, A. M.: Anal. Lett., *12*, 1063 (1979)

170. Schmitt, C. R., Cagle, G. W.: Am. Ind. Hyg. Assoc. J., *36*, 181 (1975)

171. Hackman, R. J., Rust, T.: J. Am. Ind. Hyg. Assoc., *42*, 341 (1981)

172. Genin, V. A.: Gig. Sanit., *38*, 105 (1973)

173. Burleson, G. R., Caulfield, M. J., Pollard, M.: Cancer Res., *39*, 2149 (1979)

174. Caulfield, M. J., Burleson, G. R., Pollard, M.: Cancer Res., *39*, 2155 (1979)

175. Orr, S. F. D., Sims, P., Manson, D.: J. Chem. Soc., 1337 (1956)

176. Berka, A., Korinkova, M., Barek, J.: Microchem. J., *21*, 38 (1976)

177. Barek, J., Berka, A.: Collec. Czech. Chem. Commun., *41*, 1334 (1976)

178. Barek, J., Berka, A.: Collec. Czech. Chem. Commun., *42*, 1449 (1977)

179. Dohnal, L., Zyka, J.: Microchem. J., *20*, 221 (1975)

180. Barek, J., Berka, A., Skokankova, H.: Microchem. J., *29*, 350 (1984)

181. Barek, J.: Microchem. J., *33*, in press (1986)

182. Barek, J., Berka, A., Muller, M.: Microchem. J., *33*, in press (1986)

183. Castegnaro, M., Malaveille, C., Brouet, I., Barek, J.: J. Am. Ind. Hyg. Assoc, 46, 187 (1985)

184. Klibanov, A. M., Morris, E. D.: Enzyme Microb. Technol., *3*, 119 (1981)

185. Pliss, G. B.: Vopr. Onkol., *21*, 110 (1975)

186. Mai, J.: Ber. Dtsch. Chem. Ges., *35*, 162 (1902)

187. Castegnaro, M., Barek, J., Dennis, J., Ellen, G., Klibanov, M., Lafontaine, M., Mitchum, R., van Roosmalen, P., Sansone, E. B., Sternson, L. A. Vahl, M. (eds.): Laboratory Decontamination and Destruction of Carcinogens in Laboratory Wastes: Some Aromatic Amines and 4-Nitrobiphenyl (IARC Scientific Publications No. 64), Lyon, International Agency for Research on Cancer, 1985

188. Alvarez, M., Rosen, R. T.: Int. J. Environ. Anal. Chem., *4*, 241 (1976)

189. Iovu, M., Cimpeanu, G.: Rev. Roum. Chim., *18*, 883 (1973)

190. Solomon, R. A.: US Patent No. 3,944,389 (1976)

191. Ault, E. F., Solomon, R. A.: British Patent No. 1478999 (1977)

192. Castegnaro, M., Alvarez, M., Iovu, M., Sansone, E. B., Telling, G. M., Williams, D. T. (eds.): Laboratory Decontamination and Destruction of Carcinogens in Laboratory Wastes: Some Haloethers (IARC Scientific Publications

No. 61), Lyon, International Agency for Research on Cancer, 1985

193. Castegnaro, M., Adams, J., Armour, M. A., Barek, J., Benvenuto, J., Confalonieri, C., Goff, U., Ludeman, S., Reed, D., Sansone, E. B., Telling, G. M. (eds.): Laboratory Decontamination and Destruction of Carcinogens in Laboratory Wastes: Some Antineoplastic Agents (IARC Scientific publications No. 73), Lyon, International Agency for Research on Cancer, 1985

14